Health Assessment and Physical Examination

Consulting Editor
Teresa W. Julian, Ph.D., R.N., C.S.
Adjunct Faculty and Family Nurse Practitioner
Ohio State University
College of Nursing
Columbus, Ohio

Reviewers
Cheryl Bosley, R.N., M.S.N.
Assistant Professor
Department of Nursing
Youngstown State University
Youngstown, Ohio

Linda S. Dillion, R.N., M.S.
Instructor
Baylor University
School of Nursing
Dallas-Waco, Texas

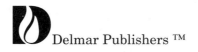

Delmar Publishers ™

I(T)P· An International Thomson Publishing Company

Albany • Bonn • Boston • Cinncinati • Detroit • London • Madrid • Melbourne
Mexico City • New York • Pacific Grove • Paris • San Francisco • Singapore • Tokyo
Toronto • Washington

Developed for Delmar Publishers Inc. by Visual Education Corporation, Princeton, New Jersey.
Publisher: David Gordon
Sponsoring Editor: Patricia Casey
Project Director: Susan J. Garver
Developmental Editor: Cynthia E. Mooney
Production Supervisor: Amy Davis
Production Assistant: Kristen Walczak
Proofreading Management: William A. Murray
Word Processing: Cynthia C. Feldner
Composition: Maxson Crandall, Lisa Evans-Skopas, Christine Osborne
Cover Designer: Paul C. Uhl, DESIGNASSOCIATES
Text Designer: Circa 86

Copyright © 1995

By Delmar Publishers
a division of International Thomson Publishing Inc.

The ITP logo is a trademark under license.

Printed in the United States of America

For more information contact:

Delmar Publishers
3 Columbia Circle, Box 15015
Albany, New York 12212-5015

International Thomson Publishing
Europe
Berkshire House 168-173
High Holborn
London, WCIV 7AA
England

Thomas Nelson Australia
102 Dodds Street
South Melbourne, 3205
Victoria, Australia

Nelson Canada
1120 Birchmont Road
Scarborough, Ontario
Canada, M1K 5G4

International Thomson Editores
Campos Eliscos 385, Piso 7
Col Polanco
11560 Mexico D F Mexico

International Thomson Publishing GmbH
Konigswinterer Strasse 418
53227 Bonn, Germany

International Thomson Publishing Asia
#05-10 Henderson Building
221 Henderson Road
Singapore 0315

International Thomson Publishing Japan
Hirakawacho Kyowa Building, 3F
2-2-1 Hirakawacho
Chiyoda-ku, Tokyo 102
Japan

1 2 3 4 5 6 7 8 9 10 XXX 01 00 99 98 97 96 95 94

Library of Congress Cataloging-in-Publication Data

Health assessment and physical examination / consulting editor, Theresa W. Julian; reviewers,
    Cheryl Bosley, Linda S. Dillion.
        p.   cm — (NSNA review series)
    Developed for Delmar Publishers Inc. by Visual Education—T.p. verso.
    ISBN 0-8273-6483-0
    1. Nursing assessment—Outlines, syllabi, etc.   2. Physical diagnosis—Outlines, syllabi, etc.
  I. Julian, Teresa W.   II. Bosley, Cheryl.   III. Dillon, Linda S.   IV. Visual Education Corporation.   V. Series.
    [DNLM: 1. Nursing Assessment—outlines.   2. Physical Examination—nurses' instruction.
  3. Physical Examination—outlines. WY 18 H4342 1995]
  RT48.H444 1995
  616.07´5—dc20
  DNLM/DLC
  for Library of Congress   94-33067
                                                                                CIP

Titles in Series

Maternal-Newborn Nursing

Pediatric Nursing

Nursing Pharmacology

Medical-Surgical Nursing

Psychiatric Nursing

Gerontologic Nursing

Health Assessment and Physical Examination

Community Health Nursing
(available in 1996)

Nutrition and Diet Therapy
(available in 1996)

Contents

Notice to the Reader...vi

Preface...vii

Chapter 1   The Interview and Health History.....................................1

Chapter 2   Types of Assessments 17

Chapter 3   Special Populations and Issues..38

Chapter 4   The Integumentary System...60

Chapter 5   The Head and Neck 76

Chapter 6   The Respiratory System 96

Chapter 7   The Cardiovascular System 117

Chapter 8   The Breasts and Axillae 136

Chapter 9   The Abdomen 149

Chapter 10 The Musculoskeletal System...163

Chapter 11 The Reproductive System...176

Chapter 12 The Nervous System..194

**Health Assessment and Physical Examination Comprehensive
Review Questions** 209

Notice to the Reader

Publisher does not warrant or guarantee any of the products described herein or perform any independent analysis in connection with any of the product information contained herein. Publisher does not assume, and expressly disclaims, any obligation to obtain and include information other than that provided to it by the manufacturer.

The reader is expressly warned to consider and adopt all safety precautions that might be indicated by the activities herein and to avoid all potential hazards. By following the instructions contained herein, the reader willingly assumes all risks in connection with such instructions.

The publisher makes no representation or warranties of any kind, including but not limited to, the warranties of fitness for particular purpose or merchantability, nor are any such representations implied with respect to the material set forth herein, and the publisher takes no responsibility with respect to such material. The publisher shall not be liable for any special, consequential, or exemplary damages resulting, in whole or part, from the readers' use of, or reliance upon, this material.

Preface

The NSNA Review Series is a multiple-volume series designed to help nursing students review course content and prepare for course tests.

Chapter elements include:

Overview—lists the main topic headings for the chapter

Nursing Highlights—gives significant nursing care concepts relevant to the chapter

Glossary—features key terms used in the chapter that are not defined within the chapter

Enhanced Outline—consists of short, concise phrases, clauses, and sentences that summarize the main topics of course content; focuses on nursing care and the nursing process; includes the following elements:
- *Client Teaching Checklists:* shaded boxes that feature important issues to discuss with clients; designed to help students prepare client education sections of nursing care plans
- *Nurse Alerts:* shaded boxes that provide information that is of critical importance to the nurse, such as danger signs or emergency measures connected with a particular condition or situation
- *Locators:* finding aids placed across the top of the page that indicate the main outline section that is being covered on a particular 2-page spread within the context of other main section heads
- *Textbook reference aids:* boxes labeled "See text pages ____," which appear in the margin next to each main head, to be used by students to list the page numbers in their textbook that cover the material presented in that section of the outline
- *Cross references:* references to other parts of the outline, which identify the relevant section of the outline by using the numbered and lettered outline levels (e.g., "same as section I,A,1,b" or "see section II,B,3")

Chapter Tests—review and reinforce chapter material through questions in a format similar to that of the National Council Licensure Examination for Registered Nurses (NCLEX-RN); answers follow the questions and contain rationales for both correct and incorrect answers

Comprehensive Test—appears at the end of the book and includes items that review material from each chapter

1

The Interview and Health History

OVERVIEW

I. **Purpose**
  A. Interview
  B. Health history

II. **The interview**
  A. Setting
  B. Structure
  C. Elements of a positive
     nurse-client relationship

D. The communication process
E. Cultural considerations
F. Sensitive topics

III. **The health history**
  A. Basic components
  B. Types of health histories
  C. Documentation

NURSING HIGHLIGHTS

1. The interview establishes a climate of support and trust. It is more than a series of questions and answers; instead, it is a conversation between nurse and client involving an exchange of information.
2. A client's beliefs about health and illness will become apparent during the interview and health history process. These beliefs affect health care.
3. Although an understanding of the health-care values of various cultures or groups is helpful, nurses should remember that persons within a culture are individually different.
4. The nurse should choose a style of communication that best suits the client and the situation. The structure of the interview and health history needs to remain flexible.
5. Clients should always be given sufficient time to think and to answer questions.
6. The nurse should remember that the interview and health history may reveal more about the client's health than the physical assessment.
7. The nurse should control, but not monopolize, the interview.

GLOSSARY

nevi—birthmarks or moles
photophobia—intolerance or sensitivity to light
polydipsia—excessive thirst
polyphagia—eating excessive amounts of food
polyuria—excessive urination

ENHANCED OUTLINE

See text pages
_____

I. Purpose

A. Interview
    1. To obtain a complete and accurate health history
    2. To obtain descriptions of symptoms and information about their development
    3. To establish a positive nurse-client relationship
    4. To guide the physical assessment process

B. Health history
    1. To provide insights into a client's current or potential health problems and his/her beliefs about health and illness
    2. To provide an organized record of a client's health as a whole, as well as any problems, needs, or concerns
        a) Serves as a baseline reference for subsequent health changes
        b) Used to develop nursing diagnoses and care plans
    3. To provide a permanent, chronologic, legal document of the examination

See text pages
_____

II. The interview

A. Setting
    1. Provide privacy.
    2. Provide freedom from excessive noise, interruptions, or distractions.
    3. Provide comfortable temperature and lighting (preferably indirect).
    4. Position furniture so that nurse and client interact at eye level.

B. Structure
    1. Introduction (initial phase)
        a) Greet client by name, including appropriate title.
        b) Introduce yourself; shake hands if you are comfortable doing so.

    c) Make the client comfortable; stay alert throughout the interview for signs of client discomfort.

    d) Explain the interview procedure and establish appropriate parameters (time frame, payment procedures, confidentiality, arrangements for future sessions).

    e) Set the tone of the interview: polite and professional.

2. Focus (working phase)

    a) Obtain health history.

    b) Avoid mechanical question-and-answer format; utilize feedback (response to 1 message affects next message).

    c) Take notes if necessary, but save most of the note taking until after the interview.

    d) Use effective communication techniques to guide the conversation (same as section II,D,1 of this chapter).

3. Termination (recapitulation and transition phase)

    a) Summarize the interview results.

    b) Establish goals and discuss follow-up plans.

    c) Ask the client if there is anything else he/she wishes to discuss before terminating the interview.

C. Elements of a positive nurse-client relationship

1. Attentiveness and sensitivity

    a) Proceed in a calm, unhurried manner.

    b) Be alert to client's anxiety or discomfort (see Nurse Alert, "Signs of Anxiety").

!   NURSE *ALERT*   !

Signs of Anxiety

Be aware of signs of anxiety that may indicate client discomfort during the interview or point to problems unrelated to the interview itself.

- Tense body posture, including facial muscles
- Dilated pupils
- Trembling
- Distended neck vessels
- Rapid or excessive talking
- Silence
- Dry mouth
- Frequent gesturing
- Rapid heart rate
- Increased blood pressure
- Sweaty palms
- Frequent sighing

       2. Acceptance
         a) Recognize own feelings and biases.
         b) Accept client; show nonjudgmental, supportive attitude.
       3. Empathy (recognizing the client's perspective)
         a) Acknowledge feelings verbally ("That sounds frightening").
         b) Express empathy nonverbally (a hand on the shoulder, nodding of head).
       4. Trust
         a) Respect confidentiality.
         b) Be honest.
           (1) Avoid statements such as "Everything's going to be all right" or "Don't be upset."
           (2) Answer questions truthfully.

    D. The communication process
      1. Effective communication techniques
        a) Open-ended questions
          (1) Used to elicit chief complaint or to begin interview process
          (2) Gives client opportunity to provide information at his/her own pace
          (3) Examples
            (a) "How have you been feeling?"
            (b) "What brought you here today?"
        b) Facilitation
          (1) Encourages the client to continue talking
          (2) Examples
            (a) Verbal, such as "Go on" or "I see"
            (b) Nonverbal, such as leaning forward or remaining silent
        c) Restatement
          (1) Rewording more specifically what client has said to enhance comprehension
          (2) Examples
            (a) Client: "I take my medication with meals."
               Nurse: "Do you mean that you take your medication before you eat?"
               Client: "No, I take my medication after I eat."
            (b) Client: "I have pain when I sit."
               Nurse: "In other words, you always have pain when you sit?"
               Client: "No, only when I sit for a long time."
        d) Reflection
          (1) Repeating what the client has said to encourage client to add more details

  (2) Examples
    (a) Client: "My arm throbs."
      Nurse: "It throbs?"
      Client: "Yes, it hurts right here."
    (b) Client: "I get dizzy sometimes."
      Nurse: "You get dizzy?"
      Client: "Yes, I get dizzy when I get up too quickly."
 e) Clarification
  (1) More direct method than restatement for understanding the meaning of client's words
  (2) Examples
    (a) "Tell me what you meant by 'a heavy feeling.'"
    (b) "You said you felt uneasy. What did you mean?"
 f) Confrontation
  (1) Presenting your observations to the client
  (2) Used when a client's comments are inconsistent or unrealistic
  (3) Examples
    (a) "You say that you don't have any pain in your arm, but I notice that you wince when you move it."
    (b) "You say you have no one who cares about you, but your son brought you here today to have treatment."
 g) Interpretation
  (1) Drawing a conclusion from the client's words or behavior: Client may confirm or deny the interpretation.
  (2) Examples
    (a) "You have many questions about possible side effects of the treatment. Are you worried about them?"
    (b) "You have a lot of complaints about the hospital staff. Do you feel they are neglecting you?"

2. Understanding nonverbal communication
 a) A client's body position, gestures, and facial expressions may give important clues to her/his psychologic state.
 b) The nurse should avoid stereotyping clients or drawing rigid conclusions based on nonverbal clues; cultural, gender, and individual differences make generalizations difficult.
  (1) Direct eye contact may indicate attentiveness and averted eyes may indicate withdrawal; in certain cultures, however, avoiding direct gaze is a sign of respect.
  (2) Although frequent gesturing can indicate anxiety, use of gestures varies among cultures and among individuals.
  (3) There are great cultural variations in the way people use space; closeness or distance to another speaker may be a function of culture rather than an indicator of psychologic state.

3. Barriers to communication (nurse)
 a) Using medical jargon or abstract language
 b) Interrupting the client

  c) Persistent questioning about something the client does not wish to discuss

  d) Making value judgments about the client's actions or beliefs

  e) Becoming defensive

  f) Asking leading questions (questions that suggest the desired answer)

   (1) Client may not answer honestly but may give an answer he/she feels the nurse will find appropriate

   (2) Examples

    (a) "You've stopped drinking, haven't you?"

    (b) "You never had a sexually transmitted disease, have you?"

  g) Offering false reassurances or using clichés

  h) Displaying anger

 4. Barriers to communication (client)

  a) Language differences

   (1) Speak clearly and concretely.

   (2) Use bilingual, culturally relevant, or language-specific questionnaires, if available.

   (3) Use a translator if necessary.

  b) Limited intelligence or level of education

   (1) Client may not be able to read or understand directions.

   (2) Questions requiring only a 1-word or 2-word answer may be helpful.

  c) Impairments or disabilities

   (1) Hearing-impaired

    (a) Use written questionnaires.

    (b) Speak slowly if the client can read lips but avoid exaggerated enunciation.

    (c) Use sign language or a translator.

   (2) Blind

    (a) Orient the client to the room.

    (b) Tell the client if anyone else is with you.

    (c) Remember to respond verbally.

 5. Developmental considerations (see sections II,A; III,A; and IV,A of Chapter 3)

  a) Infants

   (1) Obtain information from parent/legal guardian.

   (2) Observe relationship between parent/legal guardian and infant.

   (3) Refer to the infant by name.

  b) Children

   (1) Obtain information from parent or legal guardian, but direct as many questions as possible to the child.

        (2) Be aware that young children think concretely rather than abstractly.

        (3) Observe relationship between parent/legal guardian and child.

    c) Adolescents

        (1) Show an interest in the adolescent himself/herself, not just the health problem.

        (2) Discuss confidentiality.

        (3) Allow adolescent the opportunity to speak without a parent/legal guardian present.

    d) Elderly

        (1) Modify process if impairment is displayed (auditory impairment most common).

        (2) Allow additional time for client to respond.

        (3) Inquire about activities of daily living (ADLs).

E. Cultural considerations

  1. Different cultures may interpret nonverbal communication, such as touching, in different ways.

  2. Avoid making stereotypic judgments.

  3. Respect cultural, religious, and individual differences because these may affect views of health and illness; act as a nonjudgmental advocate for client.

F. Sensitive topics (e.g., sexual behavior, physical and sexual abuse, use of alcohol and substance abuse, mental illness, financial problems)

  1. If possible, ask questions after a rapport has been established (toward the end of the interview; at a later session).

  2. Discuss confidentiality.

  3. Explain why questions are relevant.

  4. Prepare client with an introductory statement such as "I'd like to ask you some questions about your sexual history."

  5. Avoid making judgments.

  6. Avoid note taking when discussing sensitive topics.

III. The health history

See text pages
_____

A. Basic components

  1. Biographic information

    a) Name, address, and phone number of client and contact person (usually relative or friend)

    b) Birthdate and sex

    c) Race, cultural background, religion: Ask specifically about beliefs or practices related to health care or diet.

    d) Marital status

    e) Social security number: for client identification

    f) Occupations (current and previous)

        (1) May indicate exposure to environmental hazards or other health hazards such as stress

        (2) May indicate socioeconomic status

      g) Birthplace: may indicate environmental health factors or cultural factors affecting health care

      h) Source of referral

      i) Source of history: usually client but may be a relative, friend, or even a stranger

      j) Reliability of information (as perceived by nurse): Note confusion, evasiveness, or inconsistencies.

2. Chief complaint or reason for seeking care

      a) Document in client's own words; use quotation marks.

      b) If client has more than 1 complaint, document complaints in order of importance (as determined by client).

3. Present illness or health status

      a) Further description of complaint or general state of health as perceived by client

      b) Investigation of symptoms (e.g., pain or other sensation)

         (1) Location: site and path of pain radiation, if any

         (2) Quality: how it feels, looks, or sounds

         (3) Quantity or severity

            (a) Degree of pain; size of lesion or rash

            (b) May use scale of 1–10

            (c) Degree of interference with ADLs

         (4) Timing or chronology: onset, duration, frequency

         (5) Setting: place, activity, person(s)

         (6) Aggravating or alleviating factors

            (a) What makes it worse? (certain movement, position, food)

            (b) What makes it better? (home or over-the-counter remedies, rest)

         (7) Associated manifestations: accompanying symptoms, often in other body systems

      c) Current medications used (frequency, amount)

4. Past status

      a) Childhood illnesses and immunizations

         (1) Information about childhood illnesses is more relevant for child's history than for adult's.

         (2) Ask adults about rheumatic fever, tetanus immunization, and hepatitis B vaccine.

         (3) Less extensive documentation is needed for the elderly, but ask if client has had polio, rheumatic fever, chicken pox; ask also about influenza and tetanus vaccinations.

      b) Accidents or traumatic injuries

         (1) Be alert to patterns of injury.

         (2) Document symptoms and treatment, including hospitalization, if any.

c) Hospitalizations
   (1) Reason for hospitalization
   (2) Treatment (include any surgical procedures, blood transfusions, and adverse reactions)
   (3) Follow-up treatment
d) Psychiatric or mental illness
   (1) Precipitating factors
   (2) Course of illness
   (3) Treatment
e) Allergies: allergens, including drugs; allergic response; treatment
f) Chronic illnesses: treatments, medications

5. Current lifestyle and psychosocial well-being
  a) Daily activities (e.g., exercise, work, leisure)
  b) Social environment (e.g., family, friends, significant others)
  c) Financial situation (e.g., housing, ability to meet health care needs for items such as food and medicine)
  d) Personal habits (e.g., smoking, alcohol or caffeine consumption, substance abuse)
  e) Nutrition (see section II of Chapter 2)
  f) Sleep patterns
    (1) Sleep and wake cycle
    (2) Difficulties falling asleep or staying asleep
  g) Developmental status (see sections II,A; III,A; and IV,A of Chapter 3)

6. Family history
  a) Immediate family members (2 generations above and 1 generation below client)
    (1) Date and cause of death
    (2) General health, including chronic diseases
    (3) May organize with genogram (family tree) showing:
      (a) Family member's relationship to client
      (b) Ages (age at death for deceased members)
      (c) Diseases, especially those that may be genetically linked
  b) Sexual partners, significant others, household members (for communicable diseases or disorders with an environmental component)

7. Review of systems
  a) Explain purpose of review—to identify potential or yet undetected disorders.
  b) Ask about symptoms (see subsequent sections); note absence as well as presence.
  c) General health: Ask about unusual symptoms, fever, chills, weight loss or gain, excessive fatigue, night sweats.
  d) Integumentary system: Ask about skin color or texture change; excessive dryness or moisture; rashes; sores; pruritis; skin growths (lesions, masses, tumors, nevi); skin disease.

  e) Head and neck
    (1) Head: Ask about headaches (frequent or severe, timing), trauma or injury, vertigo, syncope (fainting).
    (2) Eyes: Ask about last vision examination; corrective lenses; blurred vision; excessive tearing or dryness, itching, discharge; diplopia (double vision); presbyopia; myopia; photophobia; redness; pain; visual disturbances (flashes, halos around lights); glaucoma; cataracts.
    (3) Ears: Ask about last hearing examination, hearing loss, tinnitus (sensation of noise, such as ringing or buzzing, in the ear), presbycusis, infections, discharge, vertigo, pain, ear care habits.
    (4) Nose: Ask about frequent nosebleeds; frequent colds; postnasal drip; sinus infection; frequent sneezing; allergies; loss of, or impaired sense of, smell.
    (5) Mouth and throat: Ask about last dental examination, dental hygiene, bleeding gums, frequent sore throats, lesions of the mouth, changes in taste, use of dentures, difficulty swallowing, hoarseness.
    (6) Neck: Ask about pain, stiffness, masses, swelling.
  f) Gastrointestinal (GI) system: Ask about indigestion, nausea, vomiting, loss of appetite, pyrosis (heartburn), flatulence, stool color and consistency, constipation, diarrhea, abdominal pain, bowel habits, painful bowel movements, rectal bleeding, hemorrhoids.
  g) Respiratory system: Ask about history of respiratory disease, chronic cough, wheezing, shortness of breath, sputum, coughing up blood.
  h) Cardiovascular system: Ask about history of cardiovascular disease, hypertension, palpitations, chest pain, edema in extremities, heart murmur.
  i) Musculoskeletal system: Ask about pain, swelling, stiffness, muscle cramping, weakness, limitation of movement, fractures, back pain.
  j) Reproductive: Ask about history of sexually transmitted diseases (STDs); knowledge about prevention of STDs; pruritus; lesions; satisfaction with sexual activity; pain during intercourse; contraceptive practices; infertility problems; pain; swelling; masses; discharge (penile or vaginal); prostate problems, impotence (male); menstrual history and problems, date of beginning of last menstrual period, date and result of last Pap smear and mammogram, knowledge of how to perform breast self-examination, obstetric history (female).

k) Urinary system: Ask about frequency and urgency of urination; pain or burning on urination; flank pain; blood in urine; patterns of urination; change in urine flow, including retention; incontinence (inability to retain urine); history of bladder or kidney infections; history of urinary tract infections; kidney stones.

l) Nervous system: Ask about history of disease, nervousness, anxiety, seizures, syncope, tremors, tingling, numbness, sensory loss, weakness, ataxia, memory loss or forgetfulness, disorientation, difficulty with speech.

m) Endocrine system: Ask about diabetes, thyroid disease, heat or cold intolerance, polyuria, polydipsia, polyphagia, weakness.

8. Health history summary (client profile)
   a) Summary of findings
   b) Includes client's problems, strengths, and health needs

B. Types of health histories
   1. Comprehensive: obtained on initial visit
   2. Interval: taken on subsequent visits, informational update
   3. Problem-focused: information obtained about a specific problem or area
   4. Special populations: pregnant clients, infants, children, the elderly

C. Documentation
   1. Use appropriate forms and record information in ink, clearly and objectively.
   2. For every entry record the date and time; be sure client's name and identification number are on each page.
   3. Be complete but concise.
      a) Record pertinent negatives (the absence of a symptom or sign).
      b) Use words or phrases instead of sentences whenever possible.
      c) Distinguish between paraphrases of client's words and direct quotations by use of quotation marks.
   4. Use only standard abbreviations.
   5. The written record serves as a legal document.
   6. There are several types of documentation systems.
      a) Computerized records
         (1) Client-interactive (self-administered)
         (2) Practitioner-based
      b) Source-oriented records: for a particular client, separate data from each professional group (physicians' orders, laboratory reports)
      c) Problem-oriented records (POR) or problem-oriented medical records (POMR); SOAPIE format
         (1) Subjective data: history that client reports
         (2) Objective data: information obtained during physical examination
         (3) Assessment: nursing diagnosis, arrived at on the basis of subjective and objective data

I. Purpose	II. The interview	III. The health history

        (4) Plan for care of client
        (5) Implementation: nursing intervention
        (6) Evaluation: review of results

1. An important purpose of the health history is:

   a. To examine the client's cardiovascular system.

   b. To replace the physical assessment.

   c. To learn the client's beliefs about health and illness.

   d. To explain the health care system to the client.

2. "We have 30 minutes to work on your health history today. We can meet next week to complete the history and physical assessment. Our discussions and the written record are confidential." These statements would occur in which phase of the interview?

   a. Introduction or initial phase

   b. Focus or working phase

   c. Termination or recapitulation and transition phase

   d. Intervention or therapeutic phase

3. As the nurse is interviewing the client, a 16-year-old girl, the nurse notices that she answers each question very quickly, avoids direct gaze, and constantly taps her feet. The nurse has observed this client to be friendly, outgoing, and calm in other situations. This client is displaying typical signs of:

   a. Anger.

   b. Psychosis.

   c. Anxiety.

   d. Shyness.

4. As a client walks into the emergency room, the nurse asks, "Well, what's wrong with you this time?" This is an example of what type of barrier to communication?

   a. Using medical jargon

   b. Clarification of the client's perception of his/her problem

   c. Reflection of the client's words

   d. Making value judgments

5. As the nurse begins the health history, the 16-year-old client blurts out, "I think I might be pregnant! I'm so worried about telling my boyfriend!" After a period of silence, the nurse states, "I'm sure everything will work out. Don't worry about things so much, that only makes it worse. Let's finish your health history now." The nurse's response is an example of:

   a. Probing.

   b. False reassurance.

   c. Restating.

   d. Developmental interpretation.

6. During an interval health history, a first-time mother tells you her 4-month-old boy cannot finish a 4-oz bottle without periods of rest. He sleeps 23 out of 24 hours. This information may be most specifically related to a problem in which body system?

   a. Integumentary

   b. Gastrointestinal

   c. Musculoskeletal

   d. Cardiovascular

7. The family history includes which of the following areas of information?

   a. Activities of daily living (ADLs)

   b. Sleeping patterns

   c. Genogram

   d. Review of systems

8. A client's chief complaint is:

   a. Evaluation data collected by the nurse during the review of systems.

   b. Objective data recorded by the nurse.

   c. The nurse's perception of the client's problem.

   d. Documented by the nurse by quoting the client's statement of his/her health problem.

9. The nurse is completing the health history of a 45-year-old female client. She has experienced recent dizzy spells, a fainting episode, and sensations of her heart "racing and pounding." Which question about her past health status is most specifically related to her current health problem?

   a. "Have you completed the hepatitis B immunizations?"
   b. "Did you have polio as a child?"
   c. "Have you ever had rheumatic fever?"
   d. "Have you ever been hospitalized?"

10. Which of the following is the most appropriate action for the nurse who is in the process of collecting review-of-systems information?

   a. Examining each body system
   b. Documenting data in the problem oriented record (POR) format
   c. Asking, "What brought you to the clinic today?"
   d. Asking, "Have you ever experienced any numbness or tingling in your arms or legs?"

11. During the review of systems the nurse asks the client, a 57-year-old female with hypertension, "Have you experienced periods of unexplained weakness? Have you had a significant weight gain or loss?" About which body system is the nurse asking for information?

   a. Cardiovascular system
   b. Endocrine system
   c. Musculoskeletal system
   d. Gastrointestinal system

12. Based on the health history of a 44-year-old client, the nurse writes this nursing diagnosis: altered health maintenance related to excessive intake of alcohol as revealed by client. This is an example of which step in the SOAPIE format?

   a. S: Subjective data
   b. O: Objective data
   c. A: Assessment
   d. E: Evaluation

ANSWERS

1. **Correct answer is c.** Clients' beliefs about health and illness determine how they care for themselves when they are ill, how they protect their health, how they decide to seek care, and how compliant they will be with a health professional's advice. This is an important part of the health history.

   a. Examination of the cardiovascular system is part of the physical assessment.
   b. Although the health history is very important and may provide more information about the client's health than the physical assessment, the health history cannot replace the physical assessment. Integration of the health history and physical assessment is essential for an accurate, holistic assessment of the client.
   d. An explanation of the health care system is not part of the health history.

2. **Correct answer is a.** The introduction, or initial phase, includes time parameters, setting a schedule for the interview and assessment, statements about confidentiality, and introductions of the nurse and client.

   b. The focus, or working phase, includes using effective and appropriate communication techniques to collect data relevant to the health history.
   c. During the termination, or recapitulation and transition phase, the nurse summarizes the interview, discusses goals and follow-up plans, and allows time for the client to discuss any issues.
   d. Interventions, although an important part of the SOAPIE format, are not a phase of the interviewing process.

3. **Correct answer is c.** The nurse must be alert to the client's anxiety level by observing her nonverbal as well as verbal behavior.

   a. High blood pressure often has no outward behavioral symptoms.
   b. Psychotic individuals may display some of the same symptoms (although to a much

greater degree) but are also out of touch with reality.

d. Shyness is a personality trait rather than a behavioral state. The shy person is usually quiet, displays no nervous muscle movements, and maintains transient eye contact.

4. **Correct answer is d.** The nurse has already decided that the client does not have a valid complaint and expresses this in his/her response.

   a. The nurse has not used any medical jargon in her question.

   b. Clarification is a communication technique, not a barrier to communication. It involves seeking more descriptive information of the client's problem to be sure you are understanding him/her.

   c. Reflection is a communication technique, not a barrier to communication. It involves repeating the client's words to elicit more detail.

5. **Correct answer is b.** False reassurances are empty statements which may make the nurse feel better, but do little to help the client.

   a. Skillful probing, or continuing to ask questions which may make the client uncomfortable, may be necessary at times. However, most clients will react to probing by withholding information.

   c. Restating or rewording is helpful to increase the nurse's understanding of the client's statement.

   d. Developmental interpretation is drawing a conclusion based on the client's level of development.

6. **Correct answer is d.** Symptoms of fatigue when eating and excessive sleeping are 2 of the first signs of a cardiac problem in infants. The heart cannot pump enough oxygenated blood to sustain a sufficient energy level.

   a. These symptoms are not specifically indicative of problems in the integumentary system. The presence of certain lesions could indicate a problem in this system.

b. These symptoms are not specifically indicative of problems in the gastrointestinal system. Such symptoms as an increase in the frequency of bowel sounds or projectile vomiting could indicate a problem in this system.

c. These symptoms are not specifically indicative of problems in the musculoskeletal system. Such symptoms as positional deformities that cannot be manipulated into proper position or a positive Ortolani's test could indicate a problem in this system.

7. **Correct answer is c.** The genogram is a pictorial family tree that includes extended family members' relationships to the client, ages, diseases, and, for deceased members, ages at death. Various symbols are used to simplify recording.

   a, b, and **d.** ADLs, sleeping patterns, and the review of systems are important data about the client that are included in the health history, but are not part of the family history.

8. **Correct answer is d.** The chief complaint is the client's perception of his/her problem and is recorded in his/her own words.

   a. Evaluation data are collected by the nurse to determine the effectiveness of the planned interventions.

   b. The chief complaint is subjective data, or what the client states about his/her health problem.

   c. The nurse's perception of the client's problem is her/his assessment statement. This may lead to a nursing diagnosis.

9. **Correct answer is c.** Rheumatic fever in childhood can result in permanent damage to the heart's valves. Cardiovascular symptoms may not appear until adulthood.

   a and **b.** Hepatitis B immunizations and having polio as a child would not produce these symptoms.

   d. This question is a general one, not specifically related to the client's present symptoms.

10. **Correct answer is d.** Questions about tingling or numbness in the extremities identify potential problems in the client's neurologic system.

   a. Physical examination of body systems does not occur during the health history but rather during the physical assessment process.
   b. After the entire health history and physical examination are completed, documentation in the POR format is important.
   c. This question elicits data relevant to the client's chief complaint.

11. **Correct answer is b.** Reviewing the endocrine system includes assessment of the functions of the endocrine glands. Hypothyroidism, for example, could produce symptoms of weakness and weight gain.

   a, c, and **d.** Questions on weakness and weight changes together do not specifically refer to the cardiovascular, musculoskeletal, or gastrointestinal system.

12. **Correct answer is c.** The process of assessment, in which collected data are interpreted, leads to a statement of nursing diagnoses.

   a. Subjective data include direct quotes and paraphrases of what the client tells you.
   b. Objective data are measurable, such as vital signs, but are also the observations of health professionals.
   d. Evaluation is a later step in which the results of interventions are reviewed and client outcomes are viewed objectively with the purpose of trying new interventions or even revising the nursing diagnoses.

2

Types of Assessments

OVERVIEW

I. Physical assessment
  A. Approach
  B. Equipment
  C. Assessment techniques
  D. General survey
  E. Height and weight
  F. Vital signs

II. Nutritional assessment
  A. Purpose
  B. Relevant health history

  C. Assessment techniques
  D. Malnutrition classifications

III. Mental health assessment
  A. Purpose
  B. Relevant health history
  C. Assessment categories

NURSING HIGHLIGHTS

1. Properly performed, inspection can yield more information than any other physical assessment technique.
2. A physical assessment should be performed in a systematic manner, generally in a head-to-toe progression.
3. The nurse should take more than 1 body temperature measurement to gain the most accurate information.
4. Children, adolescents, pregnant or lactating women, and the elderly are at greatest risk for nutritional deficiencies.
5. The mental health assessment is a continual process that usually occurs during multiple sessions. Mental status is assessed throughout the interview and health history process.
6. The nurse should always evaluate a client's mental health status within the context of his/her culture.

GLOSSARY

antecubital—in the front of the elbow
aphasia—impaired ability or inability to use language because of brain dysfunction

ataxia—impaired muscular coordination characterized by a staggering gait and postural imbalance

Korotkoff's sounds—sounds produced by obstruction of arterial blood flow that occurs with application of a blood pressure cuff; blood pressure sounds

ENHANCED OUTLINE

I. Physical assessment

See text pages
_____

A. Approach
   1. Inform client of examination procedure at the beginning of the examination as well as during the examination.
   2. Completeness of examination may vary.
      a) Determined by client's symptoms and health history
      b) Comprehensive
         (1) To detect abnormalities
         (2) Includes general survey, vital signs, measurement of height and weight, and examination of body systems
      c) Limited: to investigate symptoms of a particular body system or region

B. Equipment
   1. Basic
      a) Thermometers
         (1) Glass-mercury (oral and rectal)
            (a) Temperature registers in 3–5 minutes (8 minutes for axillary reading)
            (b) May be less accurate than electronic thermometers
         (2) Electronic or manual digital: disposable tips for oral or rectal use
         (3) Temperature-sensitive dot, or paper-strip: disposable but less accurate than glass or electronic thermometers
         (4) Infrared aural thermometer
            (a) Electronic thermometer with blunt tip inserted into external ear; no mucous membrane contact
            (b) Records temperature in a few seconds
      b) Stethoscope: acoustic, magnetic, or electronic
      c) Sphygmomanometer: aneroid, mercury, or electronic
      d) Scales: adult, infant, bed scale
      e) Other equipment: visual acuity charts, flashlight, measuring tape, ruler, tongue depressors, cotton balls, safety pins, lubricant, disposable gloves

2. Special
   a) Ophthalmoscope
   b) Otoscope
   c) Nasal speculum
   d) Percussion or reflex hammer
   e) Tuning fork
   f) Vaginal speculum
   g) Calipers

C. Assessment techniques
   1. Inspection
      a) Begins during the interview and continues throughout the health history and physical assessment
      b) General survey (see section I,D of this chapter)
         (1) Inspect general body condition (overall health).
         (2) Compare corresponding areas: should be generally symmetric.
      c) Detailed inspection: specific areas
      d) Importance of objectivity: Nurse should avoid assumptions.
   2. Palpation
      a) Touching the body to sense tenderness; location, size, shape, consistency of organs or masses; location and character of abnormal collections of fluid; texture, moisture, temperature of skin; tremors, vibrations, spasms, movement
      b) Uses most sensitive parts of hands: finger tips (pulsation), finger pads (texture, consistency, moisture, shape), base of fingers and palmar aspect of hand (vibration), dorsal aspect (temperature)
      c) Several types (specific techniques discussed in chapters on individual systems)
         (1) Light palpation: gentle pressure, <1 cm deep
         (2) Deep palpation: increased pressure, >1 cm deep
            (a) With 1 hand
            (b) With 2 hands: bimanual palpation
         (3) Ballottement
            (a) Pressure and release; bouncing or tapping movement
            (b) Used to assess the rebound of a floating object
   3. Percussion
      a) Striking or tapping on a body surface to produce sounds or assess reflexes or tenderness
      b) Several types (specific techniques in chapters on individual systems)
         (1) Direct percussion: Lightly tap body part directly with fingers or hand.
         (2) Indirect, or bimanual, percussion: Tap finger(s) of dominant hand against finger of nondominant hand, held against the body part.
         (3) Blunt (fist) percussion
            (a) Fist is struck against body surface or against hand placed on body surface.

             (b) Blunt percussion is used to assess tenderness (especially in abdomen), not to elicit sound.

        (4) Use of percussion (reflex) hammer: to test reflexive muscle contractions (see section III,E of Chapter 12)

    4. Auscultation

      a) Listening to body sounds, movement of air or fluid

      b) Amplification of sounds with stethoscope

        (1) Chestpiece has diaphragm and bell.

          (a) Diaphragm is best for high-frequency sounds (e.g., breath sounds, friction rubs, bowel sounds).

          (b) Bell, rested lightly on skin, is best for low-frequency sounds (e.g., bruits, venous hums, third and fourth heart sounds); heavy pressure causes bell to function like a diaphragm.

        (2) Place warmed bell or diaphragm on exposed area.

        (3) Listen for sound intensity, pitch, duration, and frequency.

D. General survey: overall impression

    1. Note facial characteristics.

      a) Assess symmetry, contour, and expression.

      b) Note abnormalities: facial asymmetry, facial immobility.

    2. Note body type and stature.

      a) Assess type (e.g., ectomorph, mesomorph, endomorph).

      b) Note abnormalities (e.g., emaciation, obesity, acromegaly).

    3. Note posture and body movements.

      a) Assess posture for clues to energy level or psychologic state.

      b) Assess movements and gait for symmetry, coordination, and smoothness.

      c) Note abnormalities (e.g., slumping, hunching over; tremors; ataxia, shuffling; limping).

    4. Note dress and personal hygiene.

      a) Assess general appropriateness and ability to provide self-care.

      b) Assess personal hygiene.

      c) Note any odors.

        (1) Body: Body odor may indicate illness or high level of sweat and sebaceous gland activity.

        (2) Breath: Abnormal odors include acetone (fruity) odor or fetid odor.

    5. Assess speech.

      a) Assess clarity, tone, vocal strength, sentence structure, pace, and vocabulary.

      b) Note abnormalities (e.g., hoarseness, slurred speech, aphasia).

6. Note any signs of distress.
    a) Tense body posture, sweaty palms, or rapid speech may indicate emotional distress or pain.
    b) Shortness of breath (dyspnea), wheezing, or labored respirations may suggest cardiac or respiratory distress.
7. Note any gross abnormalities (e.g., congenital or acquired defects).
8. Assess mental status (see section III of this chapter).
9. Assess nutritional status (see section II of this chapter): well-nourished, overweight, or underweight.
10. Assess development (see Chapter 3): normal physical growth and maturation, secondary sex characteristics (adolescents).
11. Consider cultural variations.
    a) Differences in dress, behavior, and personal hygiene may reflect cultural preferences.
    b) Avoid stereotyping.
12. Document impressions.

E. Height and weight
  1. Weight
    a) Client should remove shoes and wear a gown or light clothing.
    b) Record weight to nearest ½ lb (0.2 kg).
  2. Height
    a) Use headpiece of platform scale or measuring tape.
    b) Client should remove shoes, stand straight.
    c) Record height to nearest ¼ inch (0.6 cm).

F. Vital signs (temperature, pulse, respiration, and blood pressure)
  1. Temperature
    a) Normal ranges
      (1) Normal temperature: 98.6°F (37°C), +/–1°F orally
      (2) Axillary temperature: 1°F lower than average oral
      (3) Rectal temperature: approximately 1°F higher than oral
      (4) Infants and young children up to 3 years old: average rectal temperature 99°–100°F (37.2°–37.8°C)
        (a) An infant's temperature may rise significantly (103°–105°F) with a minor infection.
        (b) With a severe infection, temperature may be normal or below normal.
      (5) Older adult: Body temperature averages about 97°F (36.1°C) but may be as low as 95°F (35°C).
    b) Procedure for taking oral temperature with glass-mercury thermometer
      (1) Shake mercury down below 96°F (35.5°C).
      (2) Place thermometer tip under tongue; have client close lips.
      (3) Remove after 5 minutes.
      (4) Client should not have consumed a hot or cold beverage or have smoked a cigarette within 15 minutes prior to taking an oral temperature.

      c) Procedure for taking rectal temperature
- (1) Select a rectal thermometer (stubby tip).
- (2) Position client lying on side (Sims's) or prone.
- (3) Lubricate thermometer and insert into anus 1 to 1½ inches (2.5–3 cm).
- (4) Hold in place for 3 minutes.
- (5) Be aware of contraindications.
  - (a) Client with bleeding hemorrhoids, lesions, or recent rectal surgery
  - (b) Client with cardiac disorder: may stimulate vagus nerve resulting in decreased heart rate
  - (c) Client with hematologic disorder such as leukemia

      d) Procedure for taking axillary temperature
- (1) Place thermometer bulb under axillary area.
- (2) Read in approximately 8 minutes.

      e) Normal variations and abnormal findings
- (1) Morning temperature: usually 2°F lower than average
- (2) Late afternoon or early evening temperature: 0.5°–1°F higher than average
- (3) Women
  - (a) Temperature generally higher than men
  - (b) Temperature slightly higher following ovulation and during the first months of pregnancy
- (4) Anxiety, dehydration, physical stress, infection, metabolic diseases: may elevate temperature
- (5) Hyperthermia: very high temperature, above 105°F (40.6°C)
- (6) Hypothermia: very low temperature, below 93°F (33.9°C)

  2. Pulse
      a) Assessment of rate, rhythm, and quality
- (1) Normal rates
  - (a) Infants: 70–190 beats per minute
  - (b) Children (see section III,B of Chapter 3 for assessment of pulse in children): Rate declines with age and varies considerably.
  - (c) Adults: 60–100 beats per minute
- (2) Rhythm: regular or irregular
- (3) Quality or amplitude
  - (a) +3: bounding (easily palpable, requires strong pressure to obliterate)
  - (b) +2: normal (palpable, not easy to obliterate with pressure)

        (c) +1: weak or thready (low volume, hard to feel, may be obliterated with light pressure)

        (d) 0: absent (not palpable)

  b) Methods

    (1) Auscultation: Listen at apex of the heart with stethoscope.

    (2) Palpation: Palpate arterial pulses (use pads of index and middle fingers).

  c) Pulse points: temporal, carotid, brachial, radial, femoral, popliteal, dorsalis pedis, and posterior tibial (see section III,G of Chapter 7)

    (1) Radial: most commonly palpated

    (2) Carotid: frequently used in emergencies

        (a) Avoid using too much pressure (may result in bradycardia).

        (b) Do not apply pressure to both carotids at the same time (may disrupt circulation to the brain).

  d) Duration: Take pulse for a full minute.

  e) Normal variations and abnormal findings

    (1) Pulse rate <60 beats per minute (bradycardia)

    (2) Pulse rate >100 beats per minute (tachycardia)

    (3) Increase in pulse rate on inspiration and decrease on expiration: sinus arrhythmia (common in children)

    (4) Pulse that fades on inspiration and strengthens on expiration: paradoxical pulse

    (5) Irregular pulse rhythm and pulse deficit: cardiac arrhythmia

    (6) Thready, weak pulse: may indicate blood loss or heart failure

3. Respiration

  a) Assess rate, depth, and rhythm.

    (1) Normal rates

        (a) Adults: 14–20 breaths per minute

        (b) Newborns: 30–60 breaths per minute

        (c) Infants and children (see sections II,B and III,B of Chapter 3): Respiration rate steadily declines with age.

        (d) Affected by such conditions as stress, trauma, disease

    (2) Character

        (a) Shallow, moderate, or deep expansion

        (b) Should be quiet and unlabored

    (3) Rhythm: should be regular (see section II,B of Chapter 3 for respiratory patterns of infants)

  b) Chest movement should be symmetrical.

  c) Recognize normal variations and abnormal findings (see section III,B,2,c,2 of Chapter 6 for additional description of respiratory abnormalities).

    (1) Irregular rhythm such as Cheyne-Stokes or Biot's breathing

    (2) Increased or decreased rate such as tachypnea or bradypnea

    (3) Unequal chest wall expansion: may indicate trauma, deformity, or collapsed lung

              (4) Use of accessory muscles: may occur in clients with chronic obstructive pulmonary disease (COPD) or respiratory distress

    4. Blood pressure (techniques may vary slightly)

      a) Systolic: force exerted on arterial walls when ventricles are contracted

      b) Diastolic: force exerted on arterial walls when ventricles are relaxed

      c) Normal findings

          (1) Adults

             (a) Systolic: 95–140 mm Hg

             (b) Diastolic: 60–90 mm Hg

          (2) Infants and children: blood pressure varies considerably and gradually increases with age

      d) Auscultatory method (listening for Korotkoff's sounds)

          (1) Place exposed arm at heart level.

          (2) Wrap sphygmomanometer cuff snugly around arm 1 inch (2.5 cm) above antecubital area.

          (3) Center cuff bladder, or arrows on cuff, over brachial artery.

          (4) Palpate brachial pulse.

          (5) Position bell or diaphragm over brachial artery.

          (6) Steadily inflate cuff to 20–30 mm Hg above point at which pulsations disappear.

          (7) Slowly open air valve, releasing pressure at approximately 2–3 mm Hg per second.

          (8) Note reading on aneroid dial or mercury column when you hear first Korotkoff's sound (systolic pressure).

          (9) Continue deflating cuff and note reading at point at which sounds become muffled (first diastolic sound) and then disappear (second diastolic sound).

        (10) Quickly deflate cuff and remove from arm.

        (11) Record systolic pressure, first diastolic sound, and second diastolic sound; some practitioners omit recording of first diastolic sound.

      e) Palpation method (used when Korotkoff's sounds are not discernable)

          (1) Apply cuff and palpate radial (or brachial) pulse.

          (2) Steadily inflate cuff to 20–30 mm Hg above point at which pulse disappears.

          (3) Release valve slowly (2–3 mm Hg per heartbeat).

          (4) Number on manometer observed with first palpable pulsation is systolic reading.

   (5) Diastolic reading difficult to obtain; may be recorded with systolic only (for example, "120/palpated").
  f) Flush method (infants): used if other methods are not possible
   (1) Apply cuff around ankle or wrist.
   (2) Wrap extremity in elastic bandage to encourage vascular emptying.
   (3) Inflate cuff to a point about 20 mm Hg above expected systolic reading (use norm table to find expected value).
   (4) Remove bandage.
   (5) Decrease cuff pressure at 2–3 mm Hg per heartbeat.
   (6) Read mean systolic-diastolic pressure at point at which vascular flush appears.
  g) Normal variations and abnormal findings
   (1) May vary (rise or fall) slightly with respiration or position changes
    (a) Decrease in systolic of less than 15 mm Hg and diastolic of less than 5 mm Hg when position changes from supine to erect: normal
    (b) Decrease of 20 mm Hg or more from supine to standing position: indicates orthostatic (postural) hypotension
   (2) Varies within a 24-hour period (circadian pattern)
    (a) Higher in afternoon and evening
    (b) Lower in late hours of sleep
   (3) Varies with physical exertion and stress
   (4) Pressure differences of 15 mm Hg between arms: may indicate cardiac disease
   (5) Readings below 95 mm Hg systolic or 60 mm Hg diastolic: may indicate hypotension
   (6) Readings above 140 mm Hg systolic and 90 mm Hg diastolic: may indicate hypertension
   (7) Pulse pressure (difference between systolic and diastolic pressure) greater than 40 mm Hg: may indicate cardiac disorder

II. Nutritional assessment

A. Purpose
 1. To identify possible malnutrition or overconsumption and its effects on the client's health
 2. To identify client's nutritional needs

B. Relevant health history
 1. Current status
  a) Has the client experienced a change in appetite or diet?
   (1) A change in dietary intake may result in nutritional deficiency and weight gain or loss.
   (2) A change in appetite may indicate disease.

See text pages

      b) Is the client experiencing significant stress or trauma?

        (1) Stress and trauma increase need for essential nutrients.

        (2) Client's eating patterns may change as a response to stress.

      c) Does the client take any medications, supplements, or appetite stimulants or depressants?

        (1) Medications can create nutritional deficiencies.

        (2) Use of vitamin and mineral supplements may indicate perceived deficiency.

        (3) Supplements may be misused.

      d) Does the client have any food allergies or chronic medical conditions?

        (1) Client may avoid certain foods because of food allergies, resulting in a nutritional deficiency.

        (2) Medical conditions

          (a) Physical problems can affect client's ability to obtain or to prepare nutritious foods.

          (b) Nutritional deficiencies are related to diseases such as AIDS, alcoholism, anorexia nervosa, cancer, and chronic obstructive pulmonary disease (COPD).

      e) Is client physically active?

        (1) Physical activity affects nutritional requirements.

        (2) Physical activity may indicate client's knowledge about health and exercise.

      f) What are the client's eating habits?

      g) Does the client's socioeconomic status allow him/her to buy sufficient amounts of food?

      h) Is the client satisfied with his/her current body weight?

  2. Past status

      a) Has the client ever had an eating disorder or substance abuse problem?

      b) Has the client dieted recently?

        (1) Ask the client to describe the diet.

        (2) Improper dieting can alter nutritional status.

      c) Has the client undergone a major illness or emotional trauma?

  3. Family history: Has anyone in the client's family been diagnosed with genetically-linked disorders such as anemia, allergies, cystic fibrosis, or obesity?

  C. Assessment techniques

    1. Anthropometric measurements

      a) Obtain baseline height and weight measurements (see section I,E of this chapter).

b) Use measurements to evaluate weight according to standard height and weight tables.
   (1) Body frame can be determined using wrist circumference measurement or elbow breadth measurement.
   (2) Further evaluate if client is 20% or more above or below standard for height and body frame size.
c) Note percentage of weight change over a certain period of time: Investigate a change in weight of more than 10% over 6 months.
d) Developmental considerations (see sections I,B; II,B; III,B; and IV,B of Chapter 3 for weight assessment of different populations)
e) Obtain skinfold measurements to determine body fat.
   (1) Triceps skinfold thickness
      (a) With client's arm flexed, find midpoint of upper arm.
      (b) Grasp client's skin between thumb and forefinger approximately 1 cm above midpoint and pull away from muscle.
      (c) Place calipers on both sides of skinfold at midpoint and release fingers slightly.
      (d) Record measurement to nearest 0.5 mm.
      (e) Repeat 1 or 2 more times.
      (f) Average the readings; refer to standard table.
   (2) Other sites for measuring skinfold thickness: subscapula, thigh, and suprailiac
f) Measure midarm muscle circumference.
   (1) Measure midpoint of upper arm (midarm circumference).
   (2) Multiply triceps skinfold thickness (cm) by 3.14.
   (3) Subtract from midarm circumference.
g) Calculate percentages of standard measurements.
   (1) Divide the actual measurement by the standard and multiply by 100.
   (2) Measurements at either extreme should be investigated.
2. Clinical examination
   a) Assess for signs of malnutrition (examples listed).
      (1) Integument: dryness, skin color changes, dull or thin hair, koilonychia (spoon-shaped nails)
      (2) Mouth: missing or loose teeth, caries, bleeding or inflamed gums, sores or fissures in lips, inflamed tongue
      (3) Eyes: pale conjunctivae, conjunctival injection (redness), dryness
      (4) Cardiovascular: tachycardia, enlarged heart
      (5) Nervous system: lethargy, decrease in ankle and knee reflexes
      (6) Musculoskeletal system: weakness, hemorrhaging, edema, wasted appearance of muscle
      (7) Gastrointestinal: liver and spleen enlargement, nausea, vomiting, diarrhea

       (8) Developmental: growth retardation

       (9) General: significant weight loss

  b) Assess for signs of obesity.

       (1) Significant weight gain over a period of time

       (2) Weight-height ratio of 20% or more above optimum weight

       (3) Body fat greater than 25% of total body weight (men) or 30% of total body weight (women)

3. Dietary analysis

  a) Record dietary intake: Ask client to recall everything consumed (food; drink; vitamin, mineral, or nutritional supplements) during a specified period (e.g., 24-hour recall, 1- to 3-days or 7- to 14-days intake record).

       (1) Type of food or drink

       (2) Amount taken

       (3) Time of day

       (4) Method of preparation

       (5) Place where food was eaten

       (6) Whether alone or with others

       (7) Why food was consumed

  b) Assess dietary intake and patterns of consumption.

       (1) Assess according to Recommended Dietary Allowances (RDAs) based on age and sex.

       (2) Assess according to food groups.

          (a) Bread, cereal, rice, and pasta

          (b) Vegetables

          (c) Fruits

          (d) Milk, yogurt, and cheese

          (e) Meat, poultry, fish, dry beans, eggs, and nuts

          (f) Fats, oils, and sweets

  c) Additional information about factors influencing food intake may be obtained from questionnaires.

4. Biochemical data analysis

  a) Total lymphocyte count (TLC): may indicate immune system function

       (1) Recognize normal range: 1500–3000/mm^3.

       (2) Below normal level may indicate malnutrition or impaired immune response.

       (3) Infections can raise level.

  b) Hemoglobin: may reflect protein status

       (1) Recognize normal ranges.

          (a) Males: 14–18 g/dl

          (b) Females: 12–16 g/dl

          (c) Children: 11–16 g/dl

(2) Above normal level may indicate dehydration.

(3) Below normal level may indicate anemia, fluid retention, or blood loss.

c) Hematocrit: measures percentage of red blood cells in blood

    (1) Recognize normal ranges.

        (a) Males: 40%–54%

        (b) Females: 37%–47%

        (c) Children: 36%–40%

    (2) Above normal level may indicate dehydration, plasma loss.

    (3) Below normal level may indicate massive or prolonged blood loss.

d) Serum albumin: aids in evaluating visceral protein stores

    (1) Recognize normal range: 3.3–5.5 g/dl.

    (2) Below normal level may indicate malnutrition.

    (3) Hydration level may affect results.

e) Serum iron

    (1) Recognize normal ranges.

        (a) Males: 70–180 mg/dl

        (b) Females: 60–160 mg/dl

    (2) Below normal level may indicate iron deficiency.

f) Serum transferrin: determines capacity of blood to transport iron

    (1) Recognize normal range: 170–390 mg/dl.

    (2) Above normal level may indicate severe iron deficiency.

    (3) Below normal level may indicate protein depletion.

    (4) Normal elevations may occur in young children and in women in the third trimester of pregnancy.

g) Total iron binding capacity (TIBC): evaluates iron storage

    (1) Recognize normal range: 250–460 mg/dl.

    (2) Above normal level may indicate iron deficiency.

    (3) Below normal level may indicate protein loss.

D. Malnutrition classifications

  1. Marasmus: characterized by depletion of fat, muscle wasting, lower than normal weight

  2. Kwashiorkor: a severe protein deficiency in which fat reserves are adequate or even excessive

  3. Marasmic kwashiorkor: condition containing elements of both disorders

III. Mental health assessment

See text pages

A. Purpose: To assess client's mental functioning

  1. Ability to function within a culture

  2. Ability to maintain social relationships

  3. Ability to maintain intimate relationships

I. Physical assessment	II. Nutritional assessment	III. Mental health assessment

B. Relevant health history
   1. Current status
      a) Is the client currently being treated for a physical or mental illness?
         (1) Onset
         (2) Treatment and progress
         (3) Medications client is taking
      b) Does the client have any concerns such as feelings of low self-esteem, anxiety, or guilt?
      c) Has the client experienced any recent mental or physical changes?
         (1) Changes in mood, behavior, memory, or ability to concentrate
         (2) Physical symptoms such as headache or tremors
      d) Does the client abuse drugs or alcohol?
      e) Is the client satisfied with family life, work, and social relationships?
      f) Where is the client's legal residence, and where is she/he living now?
   2. Past status
      a) Has the client ever been diagnosed with a mental illness?
         (1) Onset and duration
         (2) Treatment, including hospitalization

! NURSE *ALERT* !

Assessing a Client for Suicidal Tendencies

Be aware of signs that may indicate the client is considering suicide:

- Client talks about suicide.
- Client starts to give away belongings.
- Client appears very depressed.
- Client seems to have made a major decision and is suddenly at peace.
- Client has attempted suicide before.

Confronting the client with your assessment ("Are you considering suicide?") and determining if the client has the means to follow through on suicidal thoughts are crucial responses.

   b) Has the client ever suffered head trauma?
    (1) Type of injury, time of occurrence, cause of injury
    (2) Effects of injury on consciousness
   c) Has the client ever abused drugs or alcohol?
   d) Has the client ever thought of harming himself/herself or others?
    (See Nurse Alert, "Assessing a Client for Suicidal Tendencies.")
  3. Family history: Has anyone in the client's family ever been diagnosed
   with a mental illness or with alcoholism?
  4. Cultural considerations
   a) A client with a mental illness may be regarded as weak or a
    failure in many cultures.
    (1) Client may feel ashamed or guilty.
    (2) Client may experience a loss of self-esteem.
   b) Behavior and coping mechanisms vary depending on the culture.
   c) Unusual behaviors that are culturally based should not be
    considered deviant; sensitivity and understanding are crucial.

C. Assessment categories
  1. Appearance and behavior
   a) Body type: may have influence on self-esteem
   b) Body position and movement
    (1) Posture: Slouched posture may indicate depression.
    (2) Body movement: Movement should be voluntary and
     appropriate.
   c) Cleanliness, tidiness, and appropriateness of dress: Consider
    norms for age, cultural group, and lifestyle.
   d) Facial expression
    (1) Expression should be appropriate to emotions expressed.
    (2) Immobility or flatness may indicate parkinsonism or motor
     neuron weakness.
  2. Awareness and orientation
   a) Levels of consciousness
    (1) Alert and aware: normal consciousness
    (2) Obtunded, or drowsy: not fully alert or attentive
    (3) Stupor: reduced physical/mental activity, but can be aroused
     with vigorous stimuli
    (4) Comatose: completely unconscious, cannot be aroused even
     with painful stimuli
   b) Orientation: Client should be properly oriented to person, place,
    and time.
   c) Glasgow Coma Scale: used for assessment of stuporous or
    comatose clients
  3. Speech
   a) Client should exhibit speech rate, articulation, quantity, volume
    within normal ranges; responses should be appropriate.
   b) Note abnormal rate: very rapid or very slow.
   c) Note poor articulation (e.g., slurred speech, aphasia).

        d) Note poor quality of response.
          (1) Evasiveness or circumlocution
          (2) Exaggeration or confabulation

4. Attention span and memory
    a) Ask client to repeat series of random numbers (series of numbers test).
    b) Ask client to start at 100 and keep subtracting 7 (serial 7's test).
    c) Test client's ability to perform calculations indirectly by asking about client's age in a certain year or by asking the number of days, months, or years since a certain event.
    d) Test recent memory by asking client to memorize a name and address and repeat them a short time later.
    e) Observe client's response to questions and directives.

5. Thought processes
    a) Should be logical, relevant, and coherent
    b) Illogical thinking and a disconnection from reality: may indicate schizophrenia
    c) Persistent, irrational fear that results in avoidance: may suggest a phobia
    d) Repetitive actions to alleviate fear: may indicate a compulsion
    e) Repetitive, uncontrollable thoughts: may indicate an obsession
    f) A false, individual belief: may indicate a delusion

6. Abstract thinking
    a) Adult client should be able to categorize concepts and think about objects that are not physically present.
    b) Perform tests for abstract thinking.
      (1) Ask client what proverbs such as "Don't count your chickens before they're hatched" mean; evaluate responses.
      (2) Ask client to explain the similarities between 2 objects such as a chair and a sofa.
    c) Educational and cultural differences as well as language barriers may affect client's ability to demonstrate abstract thinking.

7. Judgment: Decisions should be realistic and appropriate and client should be able to meet family, work, and social responsibilities.

8. Level of insight: Client should indicate reasonable perceptions of own thoughts, behavior, and feelings.

9. Intellectual skills
    a) Assessment can provide information about intellectual abilities; however, skills are related to education and cultural background.

b) Assess in 3 areas.
  (1) General knowledge
  (2) Vocabulary
  (3) Calculation skills
10. Affect or mood
  a) Affect is the client's observable emotional state; mood is the client's subjective statements about his/her feelings.
  b) Affect or mood should be appropriate.
  c) Assess mood range: broad, restricted, flat.
  d) Note extremes such as euphoria, melancholy, or mood swings.

1. The nurse's physical and mental health assessment of the client begins:

   a. When the health history is completed.
   b. When the nurse first meets the client.
   c. After the client puts on an examination gown.
   d. After the nurse washes her/his hands.

2. A 5-year-old girl presents with an erythematous rash on her chest, back, and abdomen. After inspecting the lesions, the best way for the nurse to assess them further is to perform:

   a. Light palpation.
   b. Auscultation.
   c. Ballottement.
   d. Percussion.

3. The nurse wants to listen to the heart sounds of a 31-year-old client. She/he will use the assessment technique of:

   a. Blunt percussion.
   b. Auscultation.
   c. Inspection.
   d. Direct percussion.

4. The nurse is completing a nutritional assessment of her client, a 35-year-old man with a family history of cardiovascular disease. The nurse weighs him and measures his height. These measurements are examples of which type of nutritional assessment technique?

   a. Dietary analysis.
   b. Clinical examination.
   c. Determination of growth percentiles.
   d. Anthropometric measurement.

5. The client, a 28-year-old nullipara, is recording her morning temperature to determine her ovulation time. She telephones the nurse to discuss her monthly temperature chart. To provide her with accurate information, the nurse must know that:

   a. Morning temperatures are usually 2°F lower than average.
   b. Women's temperatures are usually higher than men's temperatures.
   c. Axillary temperatures are 1°F higher than oral temperatures.
   d. Ovulation causes a slight decrease in temperature.

6. A school nurse is assisting with sports physicals. The client, a 16-year-old, well-conditioned soccer player, arrives accompanied by his concerned mother. She states his pulse "jumps around; it's not even like mine is." The nurse takes his apical pulse while observing his respirations and finds that his pulse increases during inspiration and decreases during expiration. This condition most likely is a:

   a. Paradoxical pulse.
   b. Weak, thready pulse, +1.
   c. Rhythm irregularity and pulse deficit.
   d. Sinus arrhythmia.

7. The nurse takes a blood pressure reading on her 55-year-old male client after his breakfast. The reading is 138/104/60 mm Hg. The nurse is concerned because:

   a. The pulse pressure is 78.
   b. This blood pressure reading indicates hypotension.
   c. The systolic reading is too high.
   d. There are 3 Korotkoff's sounds in this blood pressure reading.

8. The nurse notices that her 10-year-old female client has dry, brittle hair; splitting nails; pale buccal mucosa and conjunctivae; and underdeveloped musculature. She is in the 50th percentile for height and 25th

percentile for weight. Her hemoglobin is 9 g/dl. These are clinical signs of:

a. Obesity.
b. Growth retardation.
c. Malnutrition.
d. Acromegaly.

9. The blood test that measures a client's iron stores is:

a. Hematocrit.
b. Hemoglobin.
c. Serum transferrin.
d. Total iron binding capacity (TIBC).

10. The nurse is interviewing a 33-year-old man with a history of depression. Which of the following statements alerts the nurse that he may be thinking of suicide?

a. "I have difficulty remembering tele-phone numbers and addresses. I get so confused."
b. "I have just taken a new job in Alaska. The salary is great and the weather is warm there."
c. "I was feeling in a lot of turmoil, but now I feel at peace. I've given away a lot of stuff that I won't need anymore."
d. "I'm so tired. All I want to do is sleep."

11. A nurse working in the postpartum unit has a 24-year-old client who is a Muslim and from Saudi Arabia. The client delivered a healthy baby boy yesterday. She will not answer the nurse's questions and avoids eye contact. The nurse wants to assist her with a sitz bath but she shakes her head in refusal. The nurse's best response to this situation is to:

a. Write "Client is uncooperative and re-fuses all care" in the client's chart.
b. Make flash cards with drawings for Eng-lish words.
c. Tell her supervisor that the client is showing signs of postpartum depression.
d. Investigate the norms of the client's reli-gious and cultural group.

12. The nurse's client is a 64-year-old female. The client's husband reports that his wife has been "very forgetful and confused." Which of the following questions would best help the nurse assess the accuracy of this statement?

a. "What did you have for breakfast today?"
b. "What would you do if you were in a crowded movie theater and saw a fire?"
c. "Have you ever been in treatment for a mental or emotional disorder?"
d. "How do you get along with your neighbors?"

ANSWERS

1. **Correct answer is b.** Collection of assess-ment data begins with the nurse's first in-troduction to the client. The nurse begins with inspection of the client's physical appearance, hygiene, movements, gait, demeanor, and emotional state.

   a. Assessment of the client's mental status is an integral part of the health history.
   c and d. If the nurse waits this long, she/he has missed much important data.

2. **Correct answer is a.** Palpation adds to findings observed by inspection, allowing the nurse to assess temperature, texture, and tenderness of the lesions.

   b. Auscultation is listening to the movement of air, fluid, or other body sounds, usually us-ing a stethoscope for amplification of sound. It is not used in assessing lesions.
   c. Ballottement is a specific type of palpa-tion technique involving pressure and re-lease to assess an object floating in fluid such as a fetus or the patella. It is not used in assessing lesions.
   d. Percussion is tapping on a body surface to produce sounds, determine tenderness, or assess reflexes. It is not used in assessing lesions.

3. **Correct answer is b.** Auscultation is used to listen to heart sounds. The stethoscope amplifies the sounds made by the heart.

   a. Blunt percussion or fist percussion involves striking a body area with the fist to assess tenderness, not to hear heart sounds.
   c. Inspection is visually assessing body areas for certain characteristics, such as symmetry. It cannot be used to assess heart sounds.
   d. Direct percussion is tapping a body surface directly with the fingers and cannot be used to hear heart sounds.

4. **Correct answer is d.** Anthropometric measurements are quantification studies of body size, such as height, weight, skinfold thickness, and midarm muscle circumference. These measurements can be used to determine more comparative data such as growth percentiles and percent of body fat.

   a. Dietary analysis is recording food intake for a specified period, such as 24 hours or 1 week. The nurse then assesses dietary intake in relation to Recommended Dietary Allowances for age and sex, and the amount of food within each of the food groups.
   b. Clinical examination reveals possible dietary deficiencies based on physical assessment findings. For example, multiple caries in teeth may indicate fluoride and/or calcium deficiencies.
   c. Growth percentiles are a category of anthropometric measurement used for pediatric clients.

5. **Correct answer is a.** The body's metabolic rate slows during sleep, thus causing a small decrease in body temperature.

   b. Although this is true, this datum is not relevant to the client's question.
   c. Oral temperatures more accurately reflect the body's inner core temperature since the thermometer is in contact with oral mucous membranes. The axilla is farther removed from the body's inner core; thus the axillary temperature is about 1°F lower

than the oral temperature. Also, this datum is not relevant to the client's question.
   d. Ovulation causes a slight increase in temperature.

6. **Correct answer is d.** A sinus arrhythmia is common in children and young adults. The heart rate speeds up on inspiration and slows with expiration. It can be a normal variation of pulse rhythm. Asking the client to hold his breath will stop the pulse rate from speeding up and slowing down. To rule out abnormalities, such as premature ventricular contractions, an electrocardiogram (ECG) may be done.

   a. A paradoxical pulse fades on inspiration and strengthens on expiration.
   b. A weak, thready pulse of +1 is an evaluation of pulse quality, or amplitude. The pulse is hard to feel, has low volume, fades in and out, and may be obliterated with light pressure.
   c. An irregular rhythm with a pulse deficit, or a difference between the apical pulse and the pulses of the extremities, often indicates cardiac arrhythmia. This condition is not described in the question.

7. **Correct answer is a.** The pulse pressure is the difference between the systolic and diastolic pressure. If this reading is more than 40mm Hg, a cardiac disorder may be present.

   b. Blood pressure readings below 95/60 indicate hypotension.
   c. The systolic reading is within the normal limits of 95–140 mm Hg.
   d. The presence of 3 Korotkoff's sounds in a blood pressure reading is a normal finding.

8. **Correct answer is c.** Malnutrition is manifested by but is not limited to all these clinical signs. They specifically suggest a lack of protein, iron, and calories in her diet.

   a. Criteria for obesity are a weight-height ratio of 20% or more above optimum weight or body fat greater than 25% (men) or 30% (women) of total body weight.

b. Growth retardation can be manifested by height and weight below the 3d percentile of growth charts.
d. Acromegaly is a condition caused by the excess secretion of growth hormone and is characterized by enlargement of the bones of the face, jaw, and extremities.

9. **Correct answer is d.** TIBC evaluates the body's iron storage. Readings above the normal range of 250–460 mg/dl may indicate an iron deficiency.

   a. The percentage of red blood cells in the blood is measured by the hematocrit.
   b. Hemoglobin is a conjugated protein that can carry and release oxygen.
   c. Serum transferrin is a measurement of the blood's capacity to transport iron. It is also useful in assessing visceral protein status.

10. **Correct answer is c.** Giving away personal belongings and a feeling of peace after making a decision are warning signs of suicide. Other warning signs are depression, talking about suicide, and an attempted suicide in the past.

    a. This may reflect depression, but many other conditions also interfere with memory. The statement does not suggest contemplation of suicide.
    b. This statement is an example of illogical thinking.

d. This statement could signal depression, but also could indicate a number of physical conditions such as anemia, mononucleosis, or mere lack of sleep.

11. **Correct answer is d.** Comparing a client's behavior with the norms of one's own particular culture results in ethnocentrism. Investigating the client's religious beliefs and cultural norms relative to childbirth will give the nurse insight into the client's behavior.

    a and **b.** These responses reflect ethnocentrism. The nurse has made a value judgment without collecting complete information.
    c. Postpartum depression does not usually occur 24 hours after birth, and these data are insufficient to make that assessment.

12. **Correct answer is a.** This question tests recent memory. The nurse might also ask the client to memorize a short address. Questions about remote events and computational ability might also be appropriate.

    b. This question tests judgment ability. Although judgment might also be impaired in a client with memory deficit, this question does not directly address the husband's observation.
    c. This question addresses past psychologic history, not a potential memory deficit.
    d. This question assesses social adjustment and function, not a potential memory deficit.

3

Special Populations and Issues

OVERVIEW

I. Prenatal assessment
  A. Relevant health history
  B. Physical assessment
  C. Laboratory tests and screenings

II. Neonate and infant assessments
  A. Relevant health history
  B. Physical assessment

III. Child and adolescent assessments
  A. Relevant health history
  B. Physical assessment

IV. Gerontologic assessment
  A. Relevant health history
  B. Physical assessment

V. Data analysis and diagnosis
  A. Data analysis
  B. Nursing diagnoses

NURSING HIGHLIGHTS

1. The prenatal health history is especially important as a means of identifying a high-risk pregnancy.
2. The nurse should keep in mind the emotional adjustments that affect women and their families during the pregnancy.
3. Good nutrition is an important component of a healthy pregnancy. A nutritional assessment should be done as early in the pregnancy as possible; the ideal time is before conception.
4. The nurse should remember that the assessment of the neonate provides a baseline reference for the infant's development.
5. The nurse should keep in mind that a child's health care is affected by level of parental knowledge, family cultural and religious beliefs, and parental access to health care.
6. The nurse should avoid stereotypes about the aging process; aging is affected by a variety of factors, including lifestyle, genetics, environment, and stress levels.

7. Osteoporosis occurs most frequently among postmenopausal Caucasian women and is a major cause of morbidity among the elderly.
8. Cardiovascular disease is the major cause of mortality among the elderly.

GLOSSARY

caput succedaneum—temporary swelling on presenting part of fetal head that may extend across suture lines; usually occurs during labor

chloasma—patches or spots of discolored, usually yellowish brown, skin on the face; sometimes called the "mask of pregnancy"

diastasis recti abdominis—separation of rectus muscles at abdominal midline

fetal attitude—the relationship of the fetal body parts to each other

fetal lie—the relationship of the long axis of the fetus to the long axis of the mother

fetal position—the relationship of the presenting part of the fetus to the 4 quadrants of the maternal pelvis

fetal presentation—the fetal part that first appears in the pelvis

hyperemia—increased amount of blood in a part of the body

neonate—infant from birth to 28 days of age

spider nevi—growth of dilated capillaries on skin

torticollis—neck deformity in which head is tilted to 1 side, chin to the other

ENHANCED OUTLINE

I. Prenatal assessment

See text pages
_____

A. Relevant health history
  1. Diagnosis of pregnancy
     a) Woman usually experiences signs or symptoms such as amenorrhea, breast changes, urinary frequency.
     b) Nurse may note signs such as softening of cervix or uterine isthmus, uterine enlargement, bluish discoloration of vagina.
     c) Laboratory tests (see section I,C of this chapter) can confirm pregnancy.
     d) Expected date of confinement, or expected delivery calculation (EDC): Subtract 3 months from first day of last menstrual period (LMP) and add 1 year and 7 days (Nägele's rule) or assess with ultrasonic measurement.
  2. Current status
     a) How is the client's overall health? Is the client currently experiencing any illnesses?
     b) Does the client smoke cigarettes, drink alcohol, or engage in substance abuse?

      c) What is the client's typical diet?

      d) Does the client exercise regularly?

      e) Does the client take any medications (e.g., birth control pills, seizure medication)?

      f) When was the first day of the client's last menstrual period?

      g) How does the client/client's partner feel about the pregnancy?

3. Past status

      a) Has the client ever been diagnosed with a chronic illness (e.g., diabetes, cardiovascular disease)?

      b) Has the client ever had surgery or an injury to the uterus or pelvis?

      c) Has the client ever had a miscarriage or an abortion?

      d) Has the client ever had a sexually transmitted disease (STD)?

      e) Has the client been pregnant before?

        (1) Description of pregnancy, including any complications or problems

        (2) Description of delivery, child's birth weight, description of child's overall health

4. Family history

      a) Does anyone in the client's family suffer from a chronic illness such as diabetes or cardiovascular disease?

      b) Has anyone in the client's family had multiple births?

5. Nutritional status

      a) Consider client's height/weight, dietary intake (including use of artificial sweetener, caffeine, alcohol), and activity level.

      b) Caloric requirements and nutritional needs increase, particularly for iron, calcium, and folic acid.

6. Risk factors include age under 18 or over 40; overnutrition or undernutrition; cardiovascular or renal disease or diabetes; exposure to toxic contamination; drug, alcohol, or tobacco use; bleeding after 20 weeks' gestation; multiple pregnancy; past gynecologic or reproductive problems; family disorganization, conflict about pregnancy, inadequate health care, poverty, single marital status.

B. Physical assessment

  1. Height and weight

      a) Optimal weight gain is 30–35 lb during pregnancy.

      b) Weight gain should be gradual (approximately 2–5 lb during first trimester and about 1 lb per week subsequently.

  2. Blood pressure

      a) Slight, temporary decrease during second trimester is normal; blood pressure otherwise should remain relatively unchanged.

b) Perform roll-over test at 28–32 weeks' gestation to identify women at risk for developing preeclampsia.
   (1) Take client's blood pressure with client in left lateral position.
   (2) Have client roll on back; take blood pressure immediately and again in 5 minutes.
   (3) Diastolic pressure increase of 20 mm Hg in supine position indicates positive test.
c) Pregnancy-induced hypertension may develop after the 24th week of gestation (elevation of 30 mm Hg systolic or 15 mm Hg diastolic over baseline).

3. Integumentary system
  a) Hyperpigmentation of nipples, areolae, vulva, midline of abdomen (linea nigra), and/or face (chloasma) usually fades gradually after delivery.
  b) Changes in hair quantity, texture, and oiliness may occur.
  c) Striae may appear on breasts, abdomen, buttocks, thighs; color fades over time but marks will remain.

4. Head and neck
  a) Palpate thyroid: symmetrical enlargement normal.
  b) Gum enlargement and hyperemia with bleeding may occur.
  c) Nasal congestion and nosebleeds are common.

5. Respiratory system
  a) Thoracic cage shortens and widens at base and diaphragm moves upward; maternal respiratory rate increases.
  b) Dyspnea is common in the third trimester.

6. Cardiovascular system
  a) Heart displaces slightly upward and laterally; point of maximum impulse (PMI or apical impulse) displaces laterally 1–1.5 cm.
  b) Blood volume increases 30%–50%; may result in systolic murmur.
  c) Pulse rate increases approximately 10–15 beats per minute.

7. Breasts
  a) Breasts become larger, more nodular, and may be tender; nipples are darker, larger, and more erect; Montgomery's tubercles become more prominent.
  b) Veins become more prominent due to increase in vascularity.
  c) Inspect for symmetry and color and palpate for masses.
  d) Compress nipple between index finger and thumb.
   (1) May express colostrum by 24th week of gestation
   (2) Clear to yellow, then cloudy later in pregnancy

8. Abdomen and gastrointestinal system
  a) Abdomen distends.
  b) Umbilicus may flatten or protrude; diastasis recti abdominis may occur.
  c) Peristalsis slows and bowel sounds may decrease.
  d) Uterus displaces colon laterally, upward, and posteriorly, position of appendix also changed.

e) Client may complain of heartburn or constipation.

f) Assess abdomen.

    (1) Position client with head slightly raised and knees flexed.

    (2) Inspect abdominal contour; note scars, pulsations.

    (3) Palpate abdomen to determine fundal height.

        (a) Locate uterine fundus.

            i) At 12 weeks, just above symphysis pubis

            ii) At 16 weeks, halfway between symphysis and umbilicus

            iii) At 20 weeks, at lower border of umbilicus

            iv) At 34–36 weeks, near xiphoid

        (b) Determine fundal height.

            i) Standing at supine client's right side, place palmar surface of left hand about 3–4 cm above expected fundal apex along abdominal midline.

            ii) Palpate downward with middle finger until firm, round, fundal edge is noted.

            iii) Using measuring tape, measure from top of symphysis pubis to top of fundus; measurement, in centimeters, should approximately equal number of weeks of gestation (between 22d and 36th weeks of gestation).

    (4) Palpate to determine fetal position, presentation (vertex, brow, face, shoulder, or breech), fetal lie (longitudinal, oblique, or transverse), attitude (fully flexed, poorly flexed, or extended): Leopold's maneuvers (performed after 26–28 weeks).

        (a) Client's position should be supine with knees elevated.

        (b) First maneuver determines which fetal part is in fundus; fundus is palpated with fingertips.

        (c) Second maneuver determines position of fetal back; fetus is steadied with 1 hand and palpated with the other.

        (d) Third maneuver determines which part of fetus is presenting; presenting part is palpated above symphysis with fingers.

        (e) Fourth maneuver determines how far into the pelvis the presenting part has descended; while client slowly exhales presenting part is palpated with fingers sunk deeply into pelvis above pubic bones.

g) Auscultate fetal heart.

    (1) Use Doppler instrument after 10–12 weeks and fetoscope after 16–20 weeks.

(2) Recognize normal rate: 120–160 beats per minute, slowing as pregnancy progresses.

(3) Recognize location.

    (a) At 12–20 weeks, fetal heart rate usually best heard at midline of lower abdomen, just above hairline.

    (b) After 28 weeks, fetal heart best heard over fetal back or chest.

(4) Fetal and maternal heartbeats are not synchronous.

(5) Soft, blowing sound synchronous with mother's pulse is uterine souffle (blood flowing through placenta).

9. Musculoskeletal system

  a) Pelvic joints and ligaments relax during late pregnancy.

  b) Center of gravity shifts forward, creating gait and posture changes.

10. Reproductive system

  a) Genitalia: Changes occur early in pregnancy.

    (1) Cervix softens (Goodell's sign): 4–6 weeks.

    (2) Uterine isthmus softens (Hegar's sign): 6–8 weeks.

    (3) Uterus, cervix can be flexed (McDonald's sign): 7–8 weeks.

    (4) Uterus can be palpated asymmetrically (Piskacek's sign): 7–8 weeks.

    (5) Cervix, vagina, and vulva become bluish (Chadwick's sign): 6–12 weeks.

    (6) Vaginal mucosa thickens; vaginal discharge increases.

  b) Pelvis

    (1) Pelvis may be measured at first prenatal visit to determine whether pelvic cavity will allow full-term delivery.

    (2) Measurements are repeated at 32–36 weeks (joints and ligaments have relaxed) only if pelvic cavity seems inadequate.

    (3) Recognize normal findings.

      (a) Subpubic arch: normal angle 90°

      (b) Symphysis pubis: Assess length and inclination.

      (c) Pelvic walls: normally symmetrical

      (d) Ischial spines: Assess size and prominence.

      (e) Sacrospinous notch: normal width 3–4 cm

      (f) Interspinous diameter: normal length 10.5–11 cm

      (g) Diagonal conjugate: normal length >12.5 cm

      (h) Intertuberous diameter: normal length 10.5–11 cm

C. Laboratory tests and screenings

  1. Pregnancy confirmation: Assess for presence of human chorionic gonadotropin (HCG) in urine or blood.

  2. Blood drawn at initial visit: subjected to various tests (e.g., blood type; Rh factor determination; rubella immunity; detection of HIV)

  3. Urine screening for glucose, albumin, ketones: every visit

  4. Culture of cervical discharge to diagnose gonorrhea, *Chlamydia*

5. Ultrasonography: to assess fetal size, gestational age, position; to screen for abnormalities
6. Alpha-fetoprotein (AFP): screening to detect neural tube defects; high levels in maternal blood considered abnormal and require further testing
7. Amniocentesis: analysis of amniotic fluid
8. Chorionic villus sampling (CVS): aspiration of chorionic tissue from the placental site

See text pages
_____

II. Neonate and infant assessments (up to 1 year)

A. Relevant health history: Direct questions toward parent or guardian.
   1. Prenatal history
      a) How was the mother's health during the pregnancy?
         (1) Problems or illnesses
         (2) Medications or substance abuse
         (3) Level of prenatal care
      b) How did the mother feel about her pregnancy?
   2. Labor and delivery room record (including date of birth, duration of labor, type of delivery, anesthesia or analgesia, baby's birth weight, Apgar score, vital signs)
   3. Classification
      a) Birth weight
         (1) Premature infant: <2500 g
         (2) Full term: >2500 g
      b) Gestational age (calculated from first day of last menstrual period)
         (1) Pre-term, or premature: <37 weeks
         (2) Term: 37–42 weeks
         (3) Post-term, or postmature: >42 weeks
      c) Birth weight and gestational age: weight as compared with gestational age
         (1) Small for gestational age (SGA): <10th percentile
         (2) Appropriate for gestational age (AGA): between 10th and 90th percentiles
         (3) Large for gestational age (LGA): >90th percentile
   4. Developmental status
      a) Note achievement of milestones (e.g., ability to reach for object, use thumb and forefinger to grasp small object).
      b) Use screening tests such as Denver Developmental Screening Test (DDST) to test for developmental delays from birth to age 6.

5. Nutritional status: Use growth charts to assess progress.
   a) Type (breast or bottle, introduction of solids): If mother is breastfeeding, inquire about medications she is taking.
   b) Amount and frequency
   c) Changes in or problems with feeding
6. Mental status
   a) Assess level of alertness and responsiveness.
   b) Assess parent-infant interaction: Observe parent's behavior with infant and be alert to signs of stress.

B. Physical assessment
   1. Approach: Organize examination according to infant's activity (e.g., auscultate chest if infant is sleeping) and expected responses (save potentially distressing procedures for last).
   2. General inspection
      a) Assess body proportions.
      b) Note position: neonate's limbs usually semiflexed and legs partially abducted at hip.
      c) Assess general color.
      d) Assess vital signs (see section I,F of Chapter 2 for assessment).
         (1) Temperature: rectal, aural, or axillary
         (2) Pulse: Auscultate apical pulse for a full minute.
             (a) Neonate: 140 beats per minute
             (b) 1–6 months: 130 beats per minute
             (c) 6 months–2 years: 110–115 beats per minute
         (3) Respiration: Rate varies considerably.
             (a) Neonate: 30–60 breaths per minute
             (b) 1–2 years: 20–40 breaths per minute
             (c) Respiration patterns: abdominal and nasal
         (4) Blood pressure
             (a) Norms vary greatly according to age.
             (b) Use sphygmomanometer and pediatric stethoscope/cuff.
      e) Head circumference (see section II,B,4 of this chapter)
      f) Height: Use measuring board with infant supine.
      g) Weight: Use infant scale and weigh infant nude.
   3. Integumentary system
      a) Skin
         (1) Assess color.
             (a) Caucasian neonates are reddish: Color difference from red to pale on opposite sides of body (harlequin sign) is not pathologic.
             (b) Assess for cyanosis, jaundice, or pallor.
         (2) Note birthmarks: café au lait spots, mongolian spots, hemangiomas, nevi.
         (3) Desquamation is often present at birth.
      b) Nails
         (1) Nails are usually soft.
         (2) Deviations in size and shape may indicate congenital disorder.

    c) Hair
       (1) Lanugo (downy hair, especially shoulders and back) is present in first months after birth.
       (2) Amount and texture of scalp hair varies.
  4. Head and neck
    a) Inspect and palpate head for symmetry.
       (1) Asymmetry in neonate may be due to molding of head during vaginal delivery.
       (2) Swelling and scalp discoloration that crosses suture lines may indicate caput succedaneum.
    b) Palpate anterior and posterior fontanels and cranial suture lines with infant quiet and upright and then supine.
       (1) Assess fontanels for size, shape, bulging or sunken appearance, early or late closure: Anterior fontanel normally closes 9–24 months; posterior fontanel (smaller) at 1–2 months.
       (2) Assess sutures (palpable until 6 months) for overriding of bones resulting in palpable ridges.
    c) Measure head circumference.
       (1) Assess after birth and at every examination.
       (2) Measure at greatest diameter: just above eyebrows and pinna and around occipital prominence.
       (3) Record in centimeters and plot on graph.
    d) Assess face for symmetry, feature placement, and full range of movement.
    e) Assess eyes.
       (1) Nystagmus (involuntary darting movements) and strabismus (crossed eyes) are common up to 3 months.
       (2) Inspect sclerae: Yellow sclerae may indicate jaundice, erythema may indicate hemorrhage.
       (3) Assess blink response to light stimulus.
       (4) Assess red reflex.
       (5) Assess cornea: should be smooth and transparent.
       (6) Infant should be able to fixate on and follow objects with eyes by 5–6 weeks.
    f) Assess ear placement (with inner and outer canthus of eye), symmetry, and size.
       (1) Assess auditory acuity by snapping fingers or ringing bell: Infant should respond (may blink or be startled).
       (2) Perform otoscopic exam: Pull pinna downward and insert speculum ¼–½ inch into canal; brace hand against head.

g) Assess nose placement and symmetry.
  (1) Nose of neonate is often flattened.
  (2) Assess patency of nares in neonates: Occlude 1 nostril alternately.
h) Assess mouth and throat.
  (1) Assess color; assess structure of lips, gums, tongue, hard and soft palates.
  (2) Assess reflexes: gag, extrusion.
  (3) Deciduous teeth begin to erupt at about 6 months; inspect for nursing bottle caries.
i) Assess neck.
  (1) Inspect: Webbing may indicate congenital disorder.
  (2) Palpate lymph nodes, thyroid gland, trachea, and neck muscles (mass on sternocleidomastoid muscle may indicate torticollis).
  (3) Assess head lag by holding infant's hands and slowly pulling infant from supine to sitting position.
  (4) Neck should move easily in all directions.
5. Respiratory system
  a) Inspect thorax color and shape: Infant's thorax is normally rounded and symmetrical.
  b) Assess respiration.
    (1) Abdominal, or diaphragmatic, breathing is normal; periods of apnea may occur in newborns and premature infants.
    (2) Rate varies considerably, slowing with age.
  c) Eliminate percussion: rarely performed because examiner's fingers are too large.
  d) Auscultate: Use bell or small diaphragm.
    (1) Breath sounds: louder, harsher because of thin chest wall
    (2) Abnormalities: rales, rhonchi, wheezes
6. Cardiovascular system
  a) Palpate to determine apical pulse; cardiac thrills abnormal.
  b) Auscultate: heart sounds louder, higher pitched, shorter duration than in adults; listen for extra sounds, murmurs.
7. Abdomen
  a) Inspect.
    (1) Neonate: Shape should be cylindrical; cord stump bluish white (drying agents may create bluish black color) with no signs of infection (e.g., odor, discharge, or warmth).
    (2) Older infants: Abdomen still protrudes.
  b) Auscultate for bowel and vascular sounds.
  c) Palpate.
    (1) Assess skin turgor: Crease that remains after grasping may indicate dehydration (not accurate in small-for-gestational-age [SGA] neonate).
    (2) Perform light and deep palpation: Note any tenderness, masses, or enlarged organs.
    (3) Small umbilical hernias are common.
  d) Percuss: Allow for greater amount of air in abdomen.

8. Musculoskeletal system
   a) Inspect for gross abnormalities (e.g., asymmetry, webbing of fingers, missing or extra digits).
   b) Assess joint range of motion; assess for clavicular fracture.
   c) Assess foot position: In neonate, feet may be turned inward or outward because of position in utero; examiner should be able to move foot into natural position and beyond.
   d) Assess legs: Genu varum (bowleg) is common in infancy.
   e) Assess hip joint stability: Use Ortolani's test.
9. Reproductive system: Genitalia in neonate may be swollen.
   a) Male
      (1) Foreskin: Carefully retract to inspect urinary meatus for position and discharge.
      (2) Scrotum: Palpate for descended testes, using 1 finger to block inguinal canal.
   b) Female
      (1) Separate labia majora to inspect perineal structures; note any structural abnormalities.
      (2) Bloody vaginal discharge is normal during first month.
      (3) Urethral discharge may indicate infection.
10. Anus: Check patency.
11. Nervous system
    a) Observe infant's appearance and activity for mental status, muscular function, symmetry of movement, and communication ability (crying).
    b) Assess reflexes as appropriate to age: Some reflexes disappear, others should develop.

III. Child and adolescent assessments

See text pages
_____

A. Relevant health history
   1. Approach: Speak with child and parent or guardian.
      a) Interact with child as much as possible; ask questions about behavior and social interactions.
      b) Speak honestly and directly with adolescent (11+ years old); address issue of confidentiality.
      c) Observe parent-child interaction: Be alert for evidence of stress.
   2. Current status: chief complaint or present illness
   3. Past status: prenatal, delivery, and postnatal history, including immunizations, past illness or surgery

4. Family history: to identify disorders that may have effects on a child's health
5. Developmental status
    a) Note developmental achievements; compare with children of the same age, sex, and culture.
    b) Note unusually rapid or slow development.
    c) Note age of onset of puberty.
6. Nutritional status: Inquire about diet, including snacks; food patterns and preferences; physical activity; known allergies; gastrointestinal problems; recent weight gain or loss; use of alcohol, drugs, tobacco, or caffeine; and concerns about weight.
7. Mental status
    a) Ask client (and parent or guardian of young child) about relationship with family and friends.
    b) Inquire about satisfaction with school and work, if client is employed.

B. Physical assessment: Assess most systems as for adult (see appropriate assessment sections of Chapters 5–12).
    1. Approach
        a) Be attentive with young children who may reach for instruments or fall.
        b) Provide privacy for adolescents and school-age children.
    2. General inspection
        a) Record overall impression.
        b) Record height and weight.
            (1) Measure height in centimeters or inches.
                (a) Young toddler: Measure with child in supine position.
                (b) Child who can stand unassisted: Child stands against calibrated wall measure or on platform scale with sliding head piece.
            (2) Measure weight: Weigh on platform scale lightly clothed or in a gown; if child cannot stand, weigh on infant scale.
            (3) Assess growth rate and pattern.
        c) Measure head circumference until age 2–3.
        d) Assess vital signs (see section I,F of Chapter 2 for assessment).
            (1) Temperature: axillary or aural (rectal temperatures less common because of danger of rectal perforation); oral after age 5
            (2) Pulse and respiration: Illness, exercise, emotion may increase rates.
            (3) Blood pressure: may be raised by anxiety, crying, illness
    3. Integumentary system: special considerations for prepubescent client
        a) Development of sweat and sebaceous glands during adolescence: acne common
        b) Body hair: coarse hair on face in boys; axillae and pubic areas in both sexes

4. Head and neck
   a) Eyes
      (1) Assess for strabismus in young child.
         (a) Hirschberg's test assesses location of light reflection in each eye: should be symmetrical.
         (b) Cover-uncover test assesses eye movement: any movement or drifting of eye after uncovering suggests strabismus.
      (2) Perform ophthalmoscopic examination (advanced assessment skills).
      (3) Assess visual acuity in children over 3.
         (a) Snellen's E chart can be used.
         (b) Visual acuity of 20/20 is not normally reached until age 7–8.
         (c) Lengthening of eye bulb in adolescence may bring on or worsen myopia.
   b) Ears: Inspect for position.
      (1) Limit motion of young child's head by having parent hold child or having child lie prone on examining table or parent's lap.
      (2) Correct otoscope technique is crucial to avoid ear damage.
         (a) Child under 3, pull pinna downward and out; child over 3, pull pinna upward and slightly back.
         (b) Invert otoscope; stabilize hand holding instrument against child's immobilized head.
      (3) It may be necessary to remove cerumen with irrigation or curettage.
   c) Nose: Inspect shape and symmetry, note any secretions.
      (1) Push tip of nose upward and examine interior with light.
      (2) Palpate for tenderness or deviation.
      (3) Assess patency of nares: Have client blow through nose while obstructing each naris.
   d) Face (sinuses): usually not assessed until school age
      (1) Inspect and palpate or percuss frontal and maxillary sinuses; transilluminate when sinusitis is suspected.
      (2) Sinuses widen and elongate during prepubescence; in adolescence frontal sinuses located above brows.
   e) Mouth and throat
      (1) Inspect teeth.
         (a) Examine for timing and sequence of eruption, malocclusion.
         (b) Examine for dental caries; may indicate poor nutrition, oral hygiene, or feeding practices (nursing bottle caries).

(2) Tonsils are larger in child than in adult; size peaks at about age 7.

  f) Neck: Assess neck mobility if central nervous system disease is suspected.

7. Respiratory system

  a) Inspect thorax.

    (1) Thorax shape changes at about age 7; round in younger children.

    (2) Bulging or retractions of intercostal spaces indicate respiratory distress.

    (3) Note any cyanosis or clubbing.

  b) Palpate suprasternal notch to assess trachea and identify any cardiac pulsation.

  c) Percuss: Hyperresonance is normal in young child.

  d) Auscultate: Breath sounds louder, harsher in child than in adult because of thin chest wall.

8. Cardiovascular system

  a) Palpate femoral pulse (absence or diminution may suggest aortic disorder).

  b) Auscultate heart sounds.

    (1) Heart sounds louder, of higher pitch, of shorter duration than adult's

    (2) Sinus arrhythmia normal

    (3) Splitting of S_2 during inspiration common

    (4) Point of maximum impulse (PMI or apical impulse)

      (a) Children <7: found in fourth intercostal space, left of midclavicle

      (b) Children ≥7: found in fifth intercostal space at midclavicle or slightly to the right

    (5) Murmurs

      (a) Innocent or functional: systolic; grade 3 or less in intensity; soft, low-pitched sound; occurring in more than 50% of children; absence of other evidence of cardiovascular disease

      (b) Organic: above grade 3; coarse; usually caused by acute rheumatic fever or a congenital cardiac defect

9. Abdomen

  a) Inspect shape: In toddlers shape is round and protruding with protrusion disappearing by puberty; inspect for visible peristaltic waves or hernias.

  b) Auscultate as in adult.

  c) Palpate.

    (1) Palpate lightly to detect masses, tenderness, and muscle tightness.

    (2) Palpate liver and spleen; palpate deeply for hernias, lymph nodes (kidneys usually palpable only in neonates).

    (3) If child complains of pain in an area, palpate last.

  d) Percuss boundaries of liver and spleen.

    10. Musculoskeletal system
- a) Wide-legged stance and lordosis are common until age 4.
- b) Assess spine for scoliosis: Observe from behind for deviation as child bends forward from waist with head down and arms dangling.
- c) Assess for clubfoot (talipes equinovarus): Foot should assume right angle to leg when outer/inner soles are stroked lightly.
- d) Assess muscle strength as for adult.

    11. Reproductive system: Address prepubertal and pubertal concerns and questions about sexual development and activity.
- a) Male
  - (1) Pubic hair appears at about age 12; gradually forms a diamond shape.
  - (2) Palpate scrotum, testes, and epididymis as for adult.
  - (3) Inspect penis, including foreskin and meatus.
- b) Female
  - (1) Pubic hair develops between 11 and 13: shaped like inverted triangle and usually precedes breast development.
  - (2) Inspect and externally palpate genitalia.
  - (3) Pelvic exam may be performed on adolescent female.

    12. Nervous system
- a) Observe child functioning naturally for appearance, movement, posture, and responses.
- b) Through age 6, use Denver Developmental Screening Test (DDST); after 6, assess as for adult.

See text pages

_____

IV. Gerontologic assessment: elderly (65+); old elderly (85+)

A. Relevant health history
1. Modify health history format in response to any impairments; focus on current status.
2. Perform functional assessment.
   - a) Assess ability to remain safely independent: Ask about activities of daily living (ADL).
   - b) Assess lifestyle: exercise and physical activity, sleep patterns, sexual activity, effects of drugs and illness on activities, living arrangements, stressors, typical day.
3. Assess nutritional status.
   - a) Inquire about diet, eating habits, and physical activity.
   - b) Medications may affect nutritional requirements.
   - c) Physiologic or psychosocial changes may affect appetite.

4. Assess mental health status.
   a) Assess for depression (symptoms include feelings of hopelessness, change in appetite, tiredness, thoughts of suicide).
   b) Assess self-concept: ability to cope with physical and emotional changes.
   c) Assess for adjustment to crises such as recent loss of loved one or lifestyle changes.
   d) Assess psychosocial well-being (existence of support systems, enjoyment of activities with family and friends).
5. Assess economic status: Is client able to meet daily needs?
6. Assess health habits and beliefs.

B. Physical assessment
   1. Approach
      a) Assessment is similar to that of younger adult (see appropriate assessment sections of Chapters 5–12); give special attention to physical changes that typically accompany aging.
      b) Avoid stereotyping aging client.
   2. General inspection
      a) Observe general appearance and behavior, including gait and movement.
      b) Assess vital signs (see section I,F of Chapter 2 for assessment).
         (1) Temperature may be slightly lower than in younger adult.
         (2) Pulse rate should be same as normal adult rate.
         (3) Respiration rate may be slightly higher than normal adult rate.
         (4) Blood pressure is normally higher than in younger adult: 140–160 mm Hg (systolic); 70–90 mm Hg (diastolic).
   3. Integumentary system
      a) Skin
         (1) Loss of turgor, thinning, increased dryness
         (2) Common nonpathologic lesions: cherry angiomas, seborrheic keratosis, senile lentigines; actinic keratoses may appear because of sun exposure
      b) Hair
         (1) May thin throughout body but may increase on upper lip and chin in women.
         (2) Color may change to gray, silver, or white.
      c) Nails: Growth slows; nails become thicker and may yellow, particularly toenails.
   4. Head and neck
      a) Eyes
         (1) Loss of fat within orbit, resulting in sunken appearance
         (2) Arcus senilis (opaque, gray-white ring around cornea): normal
         (3) Diminished tear production, resulting in dryness
         (4) Diminished visual acuity, especially near vision because of loss of lens elasticity

(5) Decreased peripheral vision

(6) Cataracts common

b) Ears

    (1) Hearing loss common as result of presbycusis or otosclerosis; has psychosocial effects

    (2) Changes in outer ear: coarser, stiffer cilia; cerumen accumulation (may contribute to hearing loss)

c) Nose: Sense of smell diminishes.

d) Mouth

    (1) Sense of taste declines (can contribute to altered nutrition).

    (2) Gingival recession and inflammation may occur.

    (3) Altered dentition may result from osteoporosis.

5. Respiratory system: Loss of tissue elasticity and muscle strength causes older client to be more susceptible to serious respiratory diseases; be aware of early signs of pneumonia.

6. Cardiovascular system

  a) Cardiac output decreases; heart rate may slow.

  b) Large arteries and aorta stiffen.

  c) Systolic murmurs are common.

  d) Increase in blood pressure is common: Assess for hypertension.

  e) Myocardial infarction (MI) may occur with few or vague symptoms (e.g., sudden fatigue, slight or absent chest pain, dyspnea, confusion).

7. Breasts

  a) Female

    (1) Breasts sag, become flaccid; tissue more nodular or granular.

    (2) Incidence of breast cancer increases with age: Stress importance of regular examinations, including mammogram and self-examination.

  b) Male: Gynecomastia may occur as a result of medications such as digoxin or prednisone, tumor, or diminished testosterone production.

8. Abdomen and gastrointestinal (GI) system

  a) Palpation may be easier and more accurate than in younger client due to abdominal wall thinning.

  b) Higher incidence of GI problems occurs; constipation common.

  c) Incidence of colorectal cancer increases with age.

9. Musculoskeletal system

  a) There are declines in height and muscle mass as well as reduced range of motion.

  b) Arthritic changes in joints are common: pain, stiffness, joint enlargement.

  c) Osteoporosis increases the risk of fractures (vertebrae, hip, wrist), especially in women.

10. Reproductive system
   a) Male
      (1) Testes diminish in size and firmness.
      (2) Physiologic reactions during intercourse are slower and less intense.
      (3) Benign prostatic hypertrophy common; incidence of prostate cancer increases.
      (4) Nocturnal urinary frequency or incontinence may occur.
   b) Female
      (1) Estrogen production declines.
      (2) Uterus and cervix diminish in size; vagina shortens and narrows and walls become thinner, drier.
      (3) Uterine prolapse may occur.
      (4) Nocturnal urinary frequency or incontinence may occur.
11. Nervous system
   a) Sense of touch may be diminished, especially in lower extremities.
   b) Senile tremors of head, face, or hands may occur.
   c) Reflexes diminish, some may disappear.

V. Data analysis and diagnosis

See text pages
_____

A. Data analysis
   1. Review the assessment data.
   2. Analyze and interpret the data.
      a) Recognize deviations from the norm.
      b) Identify client strengths/weaknesses, resources, teaching needs.
      c) Cluster related data; discard unrelated data.
   3. Form 1 or more tentative hypotheses (possible explanations for findings).
   4. Test hypotheses with additional assessment (physical examination, laboratory tests).
   5. Evaluate hypotheses to establish a nursing diagnosis.

B. Nursing diagnoses
   1. Definition: Clinical statements about actual or potential health problems that can be resolved, diminished, or changed by nursing intervention.
   2. NANDA nursing diagnoses
      a) Based on human response patterns of exchanging, communicating, relating, valuing, choosing, moving, perceiving, knowing, feeling
      b) Defining characteristics
         (1) Signs and symptoms
         (2) Qualifiers such as decreased, impaired, ineffective, interrupted
      c) Should follow PES (problem, etiology, signs and symptoms) format

1. The body undergoes many normal and expected physical changes during pregnancy, including:

   a. Enlargement of the heart.
   b. Deeper respirations and a decreased respiratory rate.
   c. Darkening of the areolae, nipples, and vulva.
   d. Dypsnea during the first trimester.

2. The nurse is trying to auscultate the fetal heart rate of a 23-year-old woman who is 16 weeks pregnant. To differentiate the fetal heart rate from the client's heart rate, the nurse must know that:

   a. The fetal and maternal heartbeats are synchronous.
   b. The normal fetal heart rate is 120–160 beats per minute.
   c. At this stage in pregancy, the fetal heart is usually best heard around the client's umbilicus.
   d. The uterine souffle, a soft blowing sound, is synchronous with the fetal heart rate.

3. A 16-year-old girl visits a family planning clinic to request a pregnancy test. Which of the following tests would the nurse be likely to perform?

   a. Presence of human chorionic gonadotropin (HCG) in a urine sample
   b. Presence of glucose, albumin, and ketones in a urine sample
   c. Presence of Alpha-fetoprotein (AFP) in a blood sample
   d. Chorionic villus sampling (CVS) from the placental site

4. The nurse is assisting a laboring 32-year-old woman who is 38 weeks pregnant. After 10 hours of labor, a baby boy is born. The baby's Apgar scores are 9 and 10. After mother and baby get acquainted, the nurse weighs the baby. He weighs 2700 g. Based on these data,

which of the following statements about the baby are correct?

   a. He is a premature infant and SGA.
   b. He is a full-term infant and AGA.
   c. He is a premature infant and LGA.
   d. His heart rate dropped during labor.

5. The nurse in the newborn nursery is bathing a baby girl. She notices that the baby's skin is dry and flaky. She will teach the mother that:

   a. Many babies have dry, flaky skin after birth, and losing this first layer of skin is normal.
   b. This is a reaction to lack of amniotic fluid during gestation.
   c. Using baby lotion or baby oil will help this condition.
   d. This is a reaction to soap and hospital linens.

6. Which of the following is a physical characteristic of the normal newborn?

   a. The baby is 7 days old and has not passed meconium.
   b. The baby has an asymmetrical head with overriding sutures.
   c. There is an absence of the moro reflex.
   d. Only 1 testis is present in the scrotum.

7. Every child should be screened for strabismus at every physical examination. One test for strabismus involves shining a light in both eyes and noting symmetrical placement of the light reflex in both eyes. This test is called:

   a. The corneal light reflex test.
   b. The corneal reflex test.
   c. The cover-uncover test.
   d. The extraocular eye movement test.

8. The nurse is using the otoscope to inspect the ears of a 3-year-old boy who has been crying for the last 15 minutes. The nurse finds red

tympanic membranes, visible bony landmarks, a well-defined light reflex, and mobile
tympanic membranes when a puff of air is introduced. The nurse's assessment should be:

a. Hearing deficit.

b. Middle ear infection.

c. Normal tympanic membrane.

d. Hole in the tympanic membrane.

9. The nurse is examining the musculoskeletal
system of a 3-year-old boy. Which of the following characteristics are normal in his age
group?

a. Scoliosis

b. Unequal muscle strength

c. Wide-legged stance and lordosis

d. Tibial torsion

10. The nurse is examining a 15-year-old girl.
Which of the following physical assessment
findings would be likely to cause the most
concern to the adolescent herself?

a. Dental caries in upper molars

b. Acne vulgaris

c. Snellen's eye chart screening: 20/15
in both eyes separately and both eyes
together

d. Height in the 75th percentile

11. Which of the following is an expected physical assessment finding in the elderly?

a. Substantial weight loss

b. Blood pressure of 110/70

c. Decrease in muscle mass

d. Increased skin turgor

12. After completing the health history and
physical assessment of an 87-year-old male
client, the nurse analyzes and interprets the
assessment data to identify nursing diagnoses. Which of the following nursing diagnoses is the most accurately written?

a. Suicide attempt related to ineffective
coping secondary to death of spouse

b. High risk for impaired skin integrity related to third-degree burn on palm of left
hand

c. Altered thought processes related to decreased attention span and nonreality-
based thinking

d. Total self-care deficit Level IV related to
right hemiplegia

ANSWERS

1. **Correct answer is c.** Many skin changes,
including hyperpigmentation of the nipples,
areolae, and vulva occur in pregnancy. Others include chloasma on the face and linea
nigra on the abdomen.

   a. An enlarged heart is an abnormal finding. In pregnancy the heart rate increases,
blood volume increases, and the heart is displaced upward and laterally.
   b. Respiratory depth does not significantly
increase, and respiratory rate increases.
   d. Dyspnea occurs commonly in the third
trimester.

2. **Correct answer is b.** While the normal fetal heart rate is 120–160 beats per minute,
the client's heart rate is slower at 70–100
beats per minute.

   a. The fetal and maternal heart rates cannot be synchronous because there is a significant difference in rate.
   c. At 12–20 weeks' gestation, the fetal
heart rate is best heard in the midline of
the lower abdomen, just above the pubic
hairline.
   d. The uterine souffle is caused by blood
flowing through the placenta and is synchronous with the maternal pulse.

3. **Correct answer is a.** The presence of
HCG in maternal urine or blood indicates a
positive pregnancy test and can be reliably
performed 2 days after the first missed period up to 16 weeks' gestation.

   b. During each prenatal visit, a urine sample should be checked for the abnormal presence of glucose, albumin, and ketones.
Glucose may indicate gestational diabetes.

Albumin may be present with high blood pressure and toxemia. Ketones indicate the client is not sufficiently nourished.

c. High levels of AFP in maternal blood may indicate a neural tube defect, or a problem with spinal cord development.

d. CVS involves aspiration of chorionic tissue from the placenta to detect fetal abnormalities.

4. **Correct answer is b.** A full-term pregnancy is defined as 37–42 weeks' gestation. A birth weight of 2700 grams is appropriate for gestational age (AGA).

   a. A premature or preterm infant is less than 37 weeks' gestation. A birth weight of 2700 grams at less than 37 weeks' gestation is not small for gestational age (SGA).

   c. Although he could be large for gestational age (LGA) with a birth weight of 2700 grams for a preterm gestation, he is not LGA because he is a full-term infant.

   d. The fetal heart rate may drop slightly with intense uterine contractions. Apgar scores of 9 and 10 do not support the finding that his heart rate dropped significantly during labor.

5. **Correct answer is a.** Desquamation of the first layer of skin is a normal process that begins at birth and continues for the first few weeks.

   b. Decreased amniotic fluid may be related to congenital anomalies of the fetus's renal system. There is no causal relationship between the normal process of desquamation and lack of amniotic fluid.

   c. The use of baby lotion or baby oil will make the baby's skin look better temporarily, but may irritate the skin and merely prolong the desquamation process.

   d. A contact dermatitis to soap and hospital linens usually appears as an erythematous, maculo-papular, pruritic rash.

6. **Correct answer is b.** Molding of the fetal head occurs in the birth canal, causing temporary overriding cranial sutures and an asymmetrical, elongated head in some newborns. The head returns to a more symmetrical shape as the cranial bones resume their normal positions.

   a. The passage of meconium stool usually occurs within 3–4 days after birth and indicates that the anus is patent.

   c. Newborns exhibit a strong moro reflex. This reflex involves the total body and disappears by 5 or 6 months of age.

   d. Only 1 testis or no testis may be felt in a newborn's scrotum, but this is an abnormal finding, particularly if the testes cannot be palpated in the inguinal canal. Two testes should be felt. The infant should be checked for descent of the testes at each well child visit.

7. **Correct answer is a.** The corneal light reflex test, also known as Hirschberg's test, screens for strabismus. If an eye muscle imbalance exists, the light reflex will not be symmetrically placed.

   b. The corneal reflex is tested by touching a wisp of cotton to the cornea. The eyelids should close quickly.

   c. The cover-uncover test, tests for strabismus by assessing eye movement after the cover is removed. Any movement or drifting of the covered eye is abnormal.

   d. Testing for extraocular eye movements involves moving the eyes through the 6 cardinal positions. Strabismus may be detected if both eyes do not work together well.

8. **Correct answer is c.** The presence of bony landmarks, a light reflex, and mobility of the ear drums are normal findings. The normal color of the tympanic membrane is a pearly gray; however, crying can flush the eardrum with a red color.

   a. No data support a hearing deficit.

   b. Middle ear infections are usually indicated by red, immobile tympanic membranes, no bony landmarks, and a diffuse light reflex.

   d. A hole in the tympanic membrane looks black in color.

9. **Correct answer is c.** A wide-based gait with a swayback and protuberant abdomen is normal in the toddler period.

a. Scoliosis, or curvature of the spine, is an abnormal finding and is not usually seen in the toddler age group. Scoliosis is most common in adolescent girls.
b. Unequal muscle strength is abnormal in any age group.
d. Tibial torsion, twisting of the tibia, is an abnormal finding that can occur in toddlers, preschoolers, and school-age children.

10. **Correct answer is b.** Acne vulgaris is a skin condition with comedones, papules, and pustules occurring on the face, shoulders, and back. Adolescents are extremely concerned about their appearance, and red lesions on the face will be her priority health concern.

a. Dental caries are an extremely prevalent health problem, but if the caries are in the upper molars where they are not visible, the adolescent may not be concerned about them until she has a toothache.
c. A Snellen eye screening of 20/15 in both eyes separately and together is a normal finding.
d. This adolescent girl's height is within normal limits, and she is taller than 75% of girls her age.

11. **Correct answer is c.** With aging there is a loss in muscle mass, or bulk. Muscles also become hypotonic and atrophic.

a. Weight loss does not necessarily occur. Height decreases and may decrease significantly if osteoporosis is present.

b. Blood pressure increases to 140–160 mm Hg systolic and to 70–90 mm Hg diastolic as the aorta and blood vessels lose elasticity.
d. Skin turgor decreases due to lost skin elasticity and mobility.

12. **Correct answer is a.** An accurately written nursing diagnosis contains a problem statement (or client response); and associated signs and symptoms, or defining characteristics. In this example, "suicide attempt" is the problem statement; "related to ineffective coping" is the etiology; and "secondary to death of spouse" is a defining characteristic.

b. A high risk nursing diagnosis indicates that conditions exist that are likely to develop into a problem. The etiology statement of this nursing diagnosis, a third-degree burn, indicates that the problem has already occurred. This is an actual nursing diagnosis of impaired skin integrity. No signs and symptoms are listed.
c. Altered thought processes is a valid problem statement, but the "related to" etiology statements are incorrect. Decreased attention span and nonreality-based thinking are defining characteristics of altered thought processes. A few examples of correct etiology statements for this nursing diagnosis are overstimulation, environmental overload, and insomnia.
d. Total self-care deficit, Level IV, means the client cannot participate at all in his care. In this case, he could assist because he has motor function on the left side of his body. No defining characteristics are outlined.

4

The Integumentary System

OVERVIEW

I. **Relevant health history**
   A. Current status
   B. Past status
   C. Family history

II. **Anatomy and physiology**
   A. Layers of the skin
   B. Skin appendages

III. **Assessment techniques**
   A. Approach
   B. Inspection and palpation of the skin
   C. Inspection and palpation of the hair

   D. Inspection and palpation of the nails
   E. Assessment of skin lesions

IV. **Essential nursing care for client with suspected skin cancer**
   A. Nursing assessment
   B. Nursing diagnoses
   C. Nursing implementation (intervention)
   D. Nursing evaluation

NURSING HIGHLIGHTS

1. Some changes in the skin, hair, and nails can reflect health alterations, whereas others are related to physiologic development and the aging process.
2. The nurse should compare symmetric anatomical areas throughout assessment of the integumentary system.
3. Inspection and palpation are usually performed simultaneously.
4. One of the most common types of cancer is skin cancer. It occurs most frequently, but not exclusively, in older, fair-skinned individuals.
5. The nurse should always adhere to Universal Precautions when examining skin lesions or mucous membranes.

GLOSSARY

avascular—containing few or no blood vessels
carotenemia—the presence of carotene in the blood; may produce a yellow cast to the skin

central cyanosis—bluish discoloration of the skin and mucous membranes that occurs when arterial blood has low oxygen levels, as with advanced lung disease or congenital heart defects

erythema—redness of the skin

jaundice—yellow coloring of the skin

keratin—tough protein substance in epidermis, hair, nails, and horny tissue

linea nigra—dark line extending from the umbilicus to the pubic region that occurs toward the end of the gestational period

lunula—white area near the root of the nail

melanoma—a darkly pigmented mole or tumor

peripheral cyanosis—bluish discoloration of the skin that occurs when capillaries extract excessive amounts of oxygen from venous blood, as with anxiety or exposure to cold

sclerosis—induration, or hardening, of an organ or tissue

senile lentigines—irregular areas of dark pigmentation, associated with aging

turgor—the state of normal tension in a group of cells

ENHANCED OUTLINE

I. Relevant health history

See text pages
_____

A. Current status
  1. Has the client noticed any skin, hair, or nail changes?
    a) Description (e.g., color, shape, location, other symptoms)
    b) Date of onset
    c) Suspected cause
  2. Is the client taking any medications or undergoing any treatments?
  3. Is the client experiencing any medical condition, acute or chronic illness, infection, infestation, nutritional deficiency, or emotional stress?
  4. Is the client pregnant?
    a) Skin changes can include itching, linea nigra, striae, mask of pregnancy.
    b) Hair changes can include increased growth during pregnancy and some hair loss after pregnancy.
  5. What is the client's age?
    a) Changes related to puberty include new hair growth, increased coarseness of hair, increase in size and activity of apocrine glands.
    b) Changes related to aging include graying hair, changes in hair distribution, increased wrinkling and loss of elasticity of the skin, development of senile lentigines, changes in the nails.

B. Past status
  1. Has the client had skin, hair, or nail alterations (e.g., rashes, lesions, hair loss)?
  2. Does the client have known allergies?

3. Has the client been treated for skin cancer?
   a) Type
   b) Location
4. Has the client been ill or exposed to illnesses that produce skin lesions (e.g., herpes, measles, impetigo, typhoid fever)?

C. Family history: Has anyone in the client's family been diagnosed with a skin disorder (eczema, skin cancer)?

II. Anatomy and physiology

A. Layers of the skin: epidermis, dermis, and subcutaneous tissues
   1. Epidermis: the outer layer of the skin
      a) Avascular
      b) Made up of 2 major layers
         (1) Horny layer (stratum corneum): the outermost layer
            (a) Consists of dead cells made of keratin that are shed continually
            (b) Functions
                (i) Protects against trauma and invasion by microorganisms
                (ii) Limits loss of water and electrolytes

See text pages

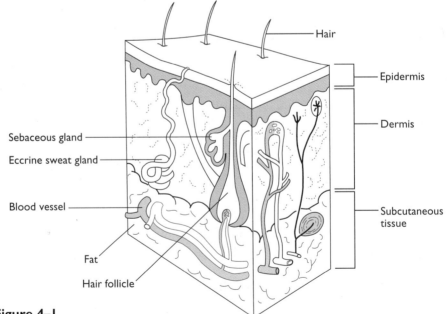

Figure 4–1
Skin Anatomy

(2) Cellular layers
    (a) Inner germinal layers
    (b) Functions
        (i) Produce keratin; replenish stratum corneum with new cells
        (ii) Produce melanin

2. Dermis: the middle layer of skin
    a) Highly vascular; contains connective tissue and blood vessels, nerves, and hair follicles
    b) Made up of 2 layers
        (1) Papillary layer
        (2) Reticular layer
    c) Functions: nourishes and supports the epidermis; provides sensory information

3. Subcutaneous tissues: lie beneath the dermis
    a) Contain mostly fat cells; may also contain some sweat glands and hair follicles
    b) Functions: insulate the body and provide energy

B. Skin appendages: sebaceous glands, sweat glands, hair, nails
  1. Sebaceous glands
    a) Appear on all skin surfaces except palms and soles of feet
    b) Produce sebum, an oily substance that is secreted into the hair follicle or onto the skin
    c) Function: Sebum lubricates and helps protect the skin.
  2. Sweat glands
    a) Eccrine glands
        (1) Open onto the skin surface
        (2) Function: help regulate body temperature
    b) Apocrine glands
        (1) Glands are located primarily in the axillary and genital areas and open onto the hair follicle.
        (2) Glands have no known function; bacteria reacts with apocrine secretions to produce body odor.
  3. Hair: consists of a shaft, follicle, and a root (or bulb), where hair develops
  4. Nails: made up of keratin
    a) Parts of the nail include the nail plate, a vascular nail bed (or matrix), a nail root, the lunula, and nail folds.
    b) Systemic illnesses may cause nail changes (see III,D,2,b).

III. Assessment techniques

A. Approach
  1. Special equipment
    a) Magnifying glass
    b) Clear flexible centimeter ruler or tape measure
    c) Flashlight
    d) Gloves

See text pages
_____

2. Environment
   a) Keep room warm.
   b) Expose only those areas being examined.
   c) Use indirect natural light or overhead fluorescent light.
3. General survey
   a) Note any irregularities (e.g., lesions, injuries, edema).
   b) Note any excessive or unusual body odor.

B. Inspection and palpation of the skin
   1. Inspect skin color.
      a) Normal findings: Skin color varies among individuals.
         (1) Normal skin color is whitish pink to brown or black.
         (2) A freckled pigmentation of the oral mucosa and a dark brown or blue gingiva may be observed in dark-skinned individuals.
         (3) Vascular flush areas include the cheeks, nose, neck, upper chest, and genital area.
         (4) Exposed areas are often darker than unexposed areas because of sun or weather damage.
         (5) The areolae and genitalia may be darker than other skin areas.
         (6) Hyperpigmentation (freckles, moles, birthmarks, mongolian spots on dark- or olive-skinned newborns, linea nigra, or the mask of pregnancy) may occur in some individuals.
         (7) The decreased pigmentation of albinism is also a normal variation in some individuals.
         (8) The skin of aging clients may be thin and translucent.
      b) Abnormal findings
         (1) Assess for cyanosis.
            (a) Cyanosis is usually most evident in the nail beds, lips, and oral mucosa.
               (i) Peripheral cyanosis appears in nail beds and is not accompanied by oral mucosa cyanosis.
               (ii) Central cyanosis appears in nail beds and in oral musosa.
            (b) Cyanosis may be difficult to detect in dark-skinned clients: Assess soles, palms, fingertips, nail beds, lips, mucosa of mouth, and palpebral conjunctiva (undersurface of the eyelids).
         (2) Assess for pallor.
            (a) Signs of pallor are most evident in the face (lips and mucous membranes) and nail beds.
            (b) Pallor may be difficult to detect in dark-skinned clients: Assess soles, palms, fingertips, and nail beds.
            (c) Pallor may indicate disease, anemia, shock, anxiety, or edema.

(3) Assess for erythema, which may be caused by a variety of conditions: heat (e.g., fever or sunburn), drug reaction, trauma, irritation, or inflammation.

(4) Assess for jaundice.

    (a) Signs of jaundice are most evident in the sclerae, palpebral conjunctiva, and lips; may also be observed under the tongue and in other skin surfaces.

    (b) Yellow pigmentation of sclerae may be normal in dark-skinned clients: Assess posterior portion of the hard palate for yellow coloring.

    (c) Jaundice may be caused by disease, severe burns, or intravenous solutions.

    (d) Yellow cast to the skin that does not involve the sclerae and mucous membranes may indicate carotenemia.

(5) Vitiligo (patchy loss of pigmentation) may indicate disease or trauma.

(6) Ecchymoses (bruises) may result from trauma or disorder.

(7) Pigmentation changes in existing skin lesions, especially moles, may indicate cancer.

(8) The appearance of new pigmented skin lesions may indicate a precancerous or cancerous condition.

    (a) Actinic keratosis: precursor to cancer
       i) Round or irregular shape
      ii) Pink, tan, gray, or red papules (see section III,E,5,a of this chapter for lesion classification)
     iii) Dry scaly surface that may itch

    (b) Kaposi's sarcoma
       i) Lesions may appear as macules, papules, plaques, or nodules (see section III,E,5,a of this chapter).
      ii) Lesions are most commonly observed on lower extremities.
     iii) Color ranges from pinkish to purplish red or reddish brown.
     iv) Condition is associated with AIDS.

2. Inspect the skin surface for moisture, edema, injuries, and lesions.

3. Palpate the skin to determine temperature, texture, turgor, and moisture content.

  a) Temperature
    (1) Assess by placing backs of fingers on skin.
    (2) Normal skin is warm to cool.
    (3) Document abnormal findings.
      (a) Hyperthermia may indicate infection.
      (b) Hypothermia may indicate shock.

  b) Texture
    (1) Assess with finger pads.
    (2) Normal skin is relatively smooth.

            (3) Document abnormal findings.

                (a) Roughness may indicate irritation or hypothyroidism.

                (b) Extreme smoothness may indicate hyperthyroidism.

        c) Turgor

            (1) Assess by picking up and releasing fold of skin.

            (2) Normal skin is elastic, although loss of turgor occurs normally with aging.

            (3) Document abnormal findings.

                (a) Loss of turgor may indicate dehydration.

                (b) Increased turgor may indicate progressive systemic sclerosis, tension, or edema.

        d) Moisture

            (1) Assess by placing backs of fingers or hands on skin.

            (2) Normal skin is dry, but varies (soles of feet, palms, and skin folds have moisture).

            (3) Document abnormal findings.

                (a) Increased perspiration may indicate pain, anxiety, or disease.

                (b) Excessive dryness may indicate dehydration or disease.

     4. Palpate any abnormal findings, such as color changes, skin lesions, vascular changes, edema, or inflammation.

   C. Inspection and palpation of the hair

     1. Quality

        a) Inspect color.

            (1) Normal hair color varies widely among individuals; gray hair is common with aging.

            (2) Document abnormal findings: Vitiligo of the scalp results in depigmentation of the hair in the affected area.

        b) Palpate texture.

            (1) Normal texture varies widely among individuals.

            (2) Document abnormal findings.

                (a) Increased silkiness and fineness may indicate hyperthyroidism.

                (b) Coarseness and dryness may indicate hypothyroidism.

                (c) Excessively oily hair may indicate hyperfunction of the sebaceous glands.

     2. Distribution

        a) Normal distribution is gender based, but distribution varies among individuals.

        b) Document abnormal findings: Abnormalities in distribution pattern (e.g., a pattern characteristic of the opposite sex) may indicate endocrine dysfunction.

3. Quantity
   a) Normal findings
      (1) Hereditary hair loss
         (a) Male pattern: usually begins in middle age with hairline recession and progresses with hair loss at the vertex, or top of the head
         (b) Female pattern: usually diffuse thinning or thinning at the frontal area with aging
      (2) Hair loss with scarring resulting in little or no hair regrowth
   b) Abnormal findings
      (1) Hirsutism (increased hair growth) may indicate disease or endocrine disorder; may also be caused by medication.
      (2) Alopecia (hair loss) may be caused by trauma, illness, infection, anxiety, starvation, endocrine dysfunction, medications, chemicals, medical treatments, or heredity.
D. Inspection and palpation of the nails
   1. Inspect color.
      a) Normal findings
         (1) Nail plate is translucent.
         (2) Lunula is white.
         (3) Nail bed is pink in light-skinned individuals and brown in dark-skinned individuals.
         (4) Longitudinal bands of darker pigment are common in dark-skinned individuals.
      b) Abnormal findings: Color changes may result from chemical exposure, trauma, infection, disease, or disorder.
         (1) Bluish color may indicate cyanosis, disease, infection, or disorder.
         (2) White spots or streaks on the nail (leukonychia) may indicate trauma, infection, disease, or poisoning.
   2. Inspect nail shape.
      a) Normal findings
         (1) Normal dorsal curvature should approximate an angle <180°.
         (2) Nails should adhere to the nail bed.
      b) Abnormal findings
         (1) Spoon nails (concave) may indicate anemia, infection, or disease.
         (2) Beau's lines (transverse indentations) may indicate disease, malnutrition, or local trauma.
         (3) Clubbing (abnormal angle of nail to nail base with spongy nail base) may indicate cardiovascular or pulmonary disease.
         (4) Dry, brittle nails may indicate malnutrition or impaired circulation.
         (5) Thickening or thinning may be related to trauma, infection, or a disorder.
   3. Apply pressure to nail plate to assess the circulation in the extremities (capillary refill time); pink color should return to nail beds within seconds after blanching.

E. Assessment of skin lesions
   1. General characteristics: size, color, shape, texture
   2. Anatomical location: body area
   3. Distribution: general or localized
   4. Pattern or configuration
      a) Discrete: separate
      b) Grouped: clustered
      c) Coalesced or confluent: merging, fused
      d) Linear: in a line
      e) Annular: in a circle
      f) Arciform: like an arc
      g) Polycyclic: more than 1 circular arrangement
      h) Reticular: in a meshed network
      i) Zosteriform (herpetiform): following a nerve route
   5. Classification: types of lesions
      a) Primary: appears on previously healthy skin because of disease or external change or irritation
         (1) Macule: flat, nonpalpable, circumscribed, <1 cm in diameter (e.g., freckles, flat mole or nevus, rubella)
         (2) Patch: flat, nonpalpable, irregular in shape, >1 cm in diameter (e.g., vitiligo, port-wine marks)
         (3) Papule: elevated, palpable, circumscribed, firm, <1 cm in diameter (e.g., wart, lichen planus, pigmented nevi)
         (4) Plaque: elevated, palpable, flat-topped, firm, >1 cm in diameter, may be coalesced papules (e.g., psoriasis, eczema)
         (5) Wheal: elevated, palpable, irregularly shaped, firm, relatively transient, variable diameter (e.g., insect bite, urticaria)
         (6) Nodule: elevated, palpable, deeper in dermis than papule, firm, 1–2 cm in diameter, may move with skin when palpated (e.g., erythema nodosum, lipomas, intradermal nevus)
         (7) Tumor: elevated, palpable, may or may not be clearly demarcated, firm, >2 cm in diameter (e.g., fibroma, neoplasms)
         (8) Vesicle: elevated, palpable, circumscribed, superficial, serous-filled, <1 cm in diameter (e.g., blister, varicella)
         (9) Pustule: elevated, palpable, superficial, similar to vesicle but filled with purulent fluid (e.g., acne, impetigo)

  (10) Cyst: elevated, palpable, encapsulated, filled with liquid or semisolid material (e.g., sebaceous cyst)

  (11) Bulla: elevated, palpable, superficial, fluid-filled, >1 cm in diameter (e.g., burn blister, poison ivy or oak blister)

 b) Secondary: results from changes in a primary lesion

  (1) Atrophy: thinning of the skin surface, loss of normal markings (e.g., striae, aging skin)

  (2) Crust: dried serum, blood, or pus (e.g., fever blister, impetigo, scab)

  (3) Erosion: loss of superficial epidermis; moist surface that does not bleed (e.g., varicella, moist area after rupture of vesicle)

  (4) Excoriation: abrasion of the epidermis (e.g., abrasion, scratch)

  (5) Fissure: linear crack from epidermis to dermis (e.g., athlete's foot, chapped skin)

  (6) Keloid: irregularly shaped, elevated, enlarged scar; more common in dark-skinned than light-skinned individuals

  (7) Lichenification: rough, thickened epidermis from irritation (e.g., atopic or chronic dermatitis)

  (8) Scale: flakes of shedding skin (e.g., psoriasis, exfoliative dermatitis)

  (9) Scar: fibrous tissue replacing injured dermis (e.g., healed wound or surgical incision)

  (10) Ulcer: loss or destruction of epidermis and dermis; concave tissue; usually scars (e.g., decubitus, stasis ulcer)

✔ CLIENT TEACHING CHECKLIST ✔

Preventing Skin Cancer

Explain the following precautions to the client:

✔ Avoid or limit sun exposure.

✔ Use sunscreen with the proper SPF (Sun Protection Factor).

✔ Be aware that some medications can increase the skin's sensitivity to sunlight.

✔ Wear protective clothing, such as a wide-brimmed hat and long-sleeved shirt.

✔ Avoid using sunlamps and tanning salons.

✔ Be aware that the sun's rays can penetrate some types of clothing.

✔ Remember that a cloudy or overcast day does not prevent sun exposure.

✔ Avoid sun exposure when the sun's rays are strongest (between 10 A.M. and 3 P.M.).

✔ Be aware of indirect sun exposure: in a pool, under an umbrella, in a car.

I. Relevant health history	II. Anatomy and physiology	III. Assessment techniques	IV. Essential nursing care for client with suspected skin cancer

See text pages

IV. Essential nursing care for client with suspected skin cancer

A. Nursing assessment
1. Gather relevant health history information (same as section I of this chapter).
2. Assess the lesion (same as section III,E of this chapter) for signs of malignant melanoma, basal cell carcinoma, or squamous cell carcinoma.
3. Assist with laboratory and diagnostic tests (biopsy, diascopy).

B. Nursing diagnoses
1. Altered health maintenance related to knowledge deficit concerning relationship between sun exposure and skin cancer
2. Knowledge deficit related to signs of skin cancer evidenced by lack of concern about lesion changes
3. Body image disturbance related to lesions on face as revealed by client's comments about own appearance
4. High risk for impaired skin integrity related to outdoor work and lack of interest in skin protection

C. Nursing implementation (intervention)
1. Help the client to identify ways to protect the skin from sun damage (see Client Teaching Checklist, "Preventing Skin Cancer").
2. Provide information on the client's medical diagnosis, treatment, and prognosis.
3. Help the client to identify coping strategies to deal with changes in appearance.
4. Encourage the client to discuss her/his feelings about the disorder.
5. Instruct the client in signs and symptoms of cancerous lesions and the importance of early detection (see Client Teaching Checklist, "Signs of Skin Cancer").

✔ CLIENT TEACHING CHECKLIST ✔

Signs of Skin Cancer

Explain the following signs of skin cancer to the client:

✔ Sore that doesn't heal
✔ Change in the shape, size, surface, sensation, or color of a wart or mole; may be accompanied by itching, scaling, oozing, bleeding, tenderness, or pain in the area
✔ Changes in skin surrounding a mole; may become pigmented, inflamed, or lose pigmentation
✔ Appearance of an unusual skin growth
✔ Change in the way skin feels

Performing a Skin Cancer Self-Examination

Explain to the client how to conduct a self-examination to assess for skin changes that may indicate cancer.

✔ Assess entire body, including the scalp, soles of the feet, and between toes, for skin changes. You may wish to have someone else inspect hard-to-see areas such as the back.
✔ Use a full-length mirror and a hand-held mirror.
✔ Use good lighting.
✔ Become familiar with your own skin so that you will be able to detect changes.
✔ Know the signs of skin cancer.
✔ Contact your doctor if you notice any unusual changes.

6. Instruct the client to assess for skin changes, particularly changes in moles (see Client Teaching Checklist, "Performing a Skin Cancer Self-Examination").
7. Offer positive reinforcement when the client takes steps toward skin protection.

D. Nursing evaluation
   1. Client demonstrates through verbalization an understanding of the signs and symptoms of skin cancer.
   2. Client demonstrates through verbalization an understanding of the importance of avoiding sun exposure.
   3. Client takes steps to minimize sun exposure.
   4. Client periodically assesses for skin changes.
   5. Client is no longer distressed about skin appearance.

1. A nurse in a family planning center has just informed a client of a positive pregnancy test. To prepare her for changes in her skin, which of the following does the nurse discuss?

   a. Erythema toxicum, milia, mottling
   b. Skin tags, dry skin, tenting
   c. Acne vulgaris, comedones
   d. Chloasma, linea nigra, striae

2. The nurse is changing an Asian infant's diaper in the newborn nursery when a new mother comes to the window. She notices that the infant's back and buttocks appear to be covered with ecchymoses. The mother wants to report the parents for child abuse. The nurse's best response to this new mother is:

   a. "I agree with you. We should report the parents right away."
   b. "Let's interview the parents first; they seem to love their baby very much."
   c. "This may look alarming to you, but this is a normal skin condition in Blacks, Asians, Hispanics, and Native Americans called Mongolian spots."
   d. "These black and blue marks will fade spontaneously in the next 2 months, so I wouldn't worry about them."

3. Spider angiomas, cherry angiomas, actinic keratoses, and poor skin turgor are more commonly found in which age group?

   a. Elderly clients
   b. Newborns
   c. Pregnant clients
   d. Adolescents

4. During the assessment of a 27-year-old female Caucasian client the nurse notes a bluish color to the client's nail beds. The client's hands are cool but inspection of the lips, buccal mucosa, and tongue reveals normal findings. These assessment findings point most directly to:

   a. Jaundice.
   b. Peripheral cyanosis.
   c. Central cyanosis.
   d. Alopecia.

5. A dirty and emaciated man is brought to the emergency room in an intoxicated state. The nurse notices purplish red plaques and nodules on his ankles and feet. The physician suspects Kaposi's sarcoma. The nurse's priority nursing action at this time is to:

   a. Assist him to the bathroom to shower.
   b. Use Universal Precautions when in contact with the client.
   c. Draw blood for an HIV test.
   d. Recommend that he call AA (Alcoholics Anonymous).

6. Palpation must be used for skin temperature, texture, turgor, and moisture assessment. To assess skin turgor, the following technique is recommended:

   a. Using the pads of the fingers, gently touch the skin in many different areas.
   b. Press 1 fingertip firmly into the skin over the client's ankle.
   c. Grasp and release a fold of skin, noting how quickly it returns to its original shape.
   d. Place the palms of the hands on the client's posterior thorax and palpate for vibrations.

7. The nurse's 82-year-old client lives in a nursing home. She usually complains of "the normal aches and pains," but today she is very tired. Her capillary refill is more than 4 seconds; her nailbeds and lips are cyanotic. These observations of her skin and nails indicate a serious problem with her:

   a. Cardiovascular system.
   b. Musculoskeletal system.
   c. Lymphatic system.
   d. Nervous system.

8. The nurse's 74-year-old client is obese and has difficulty bathing herself. While the nurse is assisting the client with her bath, the nurse notices flaky skin and red, confluent patches under her breasts, in her axillae, and between her upper inner thighs. The most appropriate nursing diagnosis is:

   a. Knowledge deficit related to skin hygiene.

   b. High risk for impaired skin integrity related to altered nutritional status, more than body requirements.

   c. Self-care deficit related to physical immobilization.

   d. Impaired skin integrity related to problems with self-care as evidenced by erythematous patches in intertriginous areas.

9. A 60-year-old woman is on the nurse's unit recovering from gall bladder surgery. During her morning care, the nurse notices a skin lesion on the back of her calf. The lesion is raised, irregular in shape, about 7 mm in diameter, and is black and brown, with a red center. The nurse's best response is to:

   a. Inform her that the skin lesion could be a malignant melanoma, a life-threatening condition, and that the physician must be notified immediately.

   b. Ask her if the lesion is itchy or bothers her.

   c. Tell her that there is a mole on the back of her leg, ask if it has changed recently, and tell her that they must call it to her physician's attention that morning.

   d. Do nothing because it is probably a benign nevus.

10. A 4-year-old girl has been enrolled in nursery school for 1 month. Her mother reports to the nurse that one morning the child awoke with focal erythema under her nose and around her mouth. Later vesicles appeared that crusted over with yellowish brown scabs. The mother reports that 4 other children at nursery school have the same lesions on their faces. These clinical findings are indicative of:

   a. Pediculosis capitis (head lice).

   b. Impetigo.

   c. Scabies.

   d. Seborrheic dermatitis.

11. A school nurse for a high school is examining a 15-year-old male client. He has come to the office complaining of "some weird stuff on my foot, and it hurts when I walk." The nurse finds 1 raised, round, rough, whitish, firm, dry, lesion about 2 mm in diameter on the ball of his left foot. The lesion is painful on palpation but is nonpruritic. It is surrounded by a callous-like ring with multiple small black spots. This assessment indicates:

   a. Verruca plantaris (plantar wart).

   b. Tinea pedis (athlete's foot).

   c. Eczema.

   d. Vitiligo.

12. A 33-year-old female client is planning a trip to Mexico 1 month from now. She asks how she can best prepare her skin for the intense sunshine in June. She wishes to "get a good tan" but does not wish to burn. The nurse's best advice is:

   a. "Use a tanning bed once a week for 4 weeks before departure."

   b. "Expose your skin to natural sunlight every day from 1 P.M.–1:30 P.M. until departure."

   c. "Try to get a base tan during cloudy days."

   d. "Pack sun block, sunglasses, wide-brimmed hats, long-sleeved shirts, and long pants to protect yourself from the sun."

ANSWERS

---

1. Correct answer is d. Skin changes that may occur during pregnancy include chloasma, brownish colorations around the eyes and cheeks known as the mask of pregnancy; the appearance of linea nigra, a dark longitudinal line down the midline of the abdomen; striae, or stretch marks, as the abdomen expands.

   a. Erythema toxicum, milia, and mottling are skin conditions associated with newborns.

b. Skin tags, dry skin, and tenting are common skin conditions in the elderly.

c. Acne vulgaris and comedones are seen more frequently in adolescents, although pregnancy can increase the oiliness of the skin and exacerbate acne.

2. **Correct answer is c.** Mongolian spots look like bruises, but are not the result of trauma. They are a benign skin condition common in nonwhite populations and fade spontaneously.

a and **b.** These remarks are inappropriate nursing actions based on data given in the situation and the expected knowledge base of nurse.

d. The marks will fade spontaneously, but this statement does not address the new mother's concern and implies that the marks are bruises.

3. **Correct answer is a.** Elderly clients more commonly have spider angiomas, cherry angiomas, actinic keratoses, and poor skin turgor.

b and **d.** Newborns and adolescents normally have good skin turgor and do not exhibit these skin lesions.

c. Pregnant clients normally have good skin turgor. They may have spider angiomas but typically have none of the other lesions.

4. **Correct answer is b.** Peripheral cyanosis causes a bluish color in the client's nail beds and cool skin temperature without cyanosis of the lips, buccal mucosa, or tongue.

a. Jaundice, which may indicate liver dysfunction, causes a yellowish cast first to the sclera and then to the mucous membranes and skin.

c. A client with central cyanosis would show bluish coloring in the lips, buccal mucosa, or tongue.

d. Alopecia is hair loss on the scalp or body.

5. **Correct answer is b.** Implementation of Universal Precautions is the priority nursing action before anything else is considered.

Universal Precautions to protect oneself and the client from the spread of disease should be used in all client care situations, not just when AIDS may be suspected.

a. Showering while intoxicated may be dangerous, and data do not support this as a priority need at this time.

c. An HIV test may be ordered later, but this is not the priority at this time.

d. This is not an appropriate nursing action at this time. The client should be in an alert and sober mental state before AA is discussed.

6. **Correct answer is c.** Skin turgor refers to the mobility, hydration, and elasticity of the skin and underlying tissues. Grasping a fold of skin, pulling upward, and timing its return to its normal shape tells us the degree of skin turgor. It is best done on the anterior chest. Normal skin will resume its shape immediately. The skin returns to its normal shape very slowly in elderly clients and premature infants. It is 1 indicator of the client's hydration status.

a. This technique may be used to assess skin texture. Gloves may be worn to protect you and the client, but tactile sensitivity will be reduced.

b. This technique may be used to assess ankle edema. Observe if the skin resumes its normal shape or appears "pitted," indicating a large accumulation of fluid.

d. This technique is part of the assessment for tactile fremitus, performed to assess the contents of the lungs by palpating voice vibrations on the chest and back.

7. **Correct answer is a.** The color of the lips and nailbeds reflects the degree of oxygenation of blood and the effectiveness of the heart as a pump to circulate the oxygenated blood. Cyanosis, a blue color to her lips and nailbeds, may indicate a problem with her respiratory or cardiovascular systems. Capillary refill of more than 4 seconds indicates a circulatory problem.

b, c, and **d.** Cyanotic lips and nailbeds do not directly indicate dysfunctions of the musculoskeletal, lymphatic, or nervous systems. However, dysfunctions of these systems may occur as a result of cardiac or respiratory failure.

8. **Correct answer is d.** Her skin integrity is compromised as evidenced by the reddened, macerated areas in the skin folds of her body. Based on the data given, her problem is related to the difficulty she has bathing herself.

   a. The information given does not support a knowledge deficit of this type.
   b. Her obesity reflects an altered nutritional state, but she is not at high risk for impaired skin integrity because skin maceration and exfoliation damage have already occurred.
   c. She has a self-care deficit, but data given reveal nothing about physical immobilization.

9. **Correct answer is c.** The skin lesion meets the ABCD criteria for malignant melanoma and must be reported to the physician. The client should be made aware of the lesion and additional data, such as recent changes, should be collected.

   a. The client should not be unduly alarmed by the possibility of a malignant disease until the data are confirmed.
   b. These additional data are useful, but the priority reponse is to inform the physician about the condition.
   d. This skin lesion is probably not a benign nevus. It may not be malignant melanoma, but it may be a dysplastic nevus.

10. **Correct answer is b.** Impetigo is a highly contagious skin condition that erupts in moist areas around the nose and mouth.

    a. Head lice are detected by the presence of tiny white nits (eggs) attached to the hair shaft.

    c. Scabies is caused by a mite that burrows under the skin, leaving red, itchy papules and excoriations that most commonly appear on the hands, wrists, thighs, genitalia, axillae, or around the waist.
    d. Seborrheic dermatitis is an inflammatory skin disease manifested by red papules and pustules usually appearing on oily, flaky skin of the scalp and face.

11. **Correct answer is a.** A plantar wart occurs on the plantar surface of the feet, may grow to the point of causing pain when walking, is spread by satellite lesions, and may resemble a callus in appearance.

    b. Vesicles and red, moist fissures between the toes accompanied by an itchy, burning sensation indicate athelete's foot.
    c. Eczema is a superficial dermatitis with reddened areas of skin and may involve vesicles and crusts.
    d. Vitiligo is the absence of skin pigment, resulting in white, irregular patches. Vitiligo typically occurs on the dorsal surface of the hands but may occur on any pigmented skin area.

12. **Correct answer is d.** There is no safe level of sun exposure. The skin should be protected from the sun at all times. Sunburn and frequent tanning increase the risk of skin cancer.

    a. Tanning beds still expose the body to damaging ultraviolet light and can cause severe burning.
    b. Exposure to sunlight should be avoided especially during the hours of 10 A.M.–3 P.M., when the rays are most direct and intense.
    c. Clouds do not protect the skin from ultraviolet light.

5

The Head and Neck

OVERVIEW

I. Relevant health history
   A. Current status
   B. Past status
   C. Family history

II. Anatomy and physiology
   A. The head and neck
   B. The eye
   C. The ear
   D. The nose
   E. The mouth and oropharynx

III. Assessment techniques
   A. Approach
   B. Inspection and palpation of the head
   C. Inspection, palpation, and auscultation of the face
   D. Inspection, palpation, and auscultation of the neck

   E. Inspection and palpation of the eye
   F. Inspection and palpation of the ear
   G. Inspection and palpation of the nose
   H. Palpation, percussion, and transillumination of the frontal and maxillary sinuses
   I. Inspection and palpation of the mouth

IV. Essential nursing care for client with neck pain
   A. Nursing assessment
   B. Nursing diagnoses
   C. Nursing implementation (intervention)
   D. Nursing evaluation

NURSING HIGHLIGHTS

1. The nurse should keep in mind that most headaches are nonpathologic but that some indicate serious health problems.
2. The ear, nose, and throat assessment reveals information about the respiratory and digestive systems.
3. The eye assessment can reveal important information about systemic health.

hydrocephaly—increased accumulation of cerebrospinal fluid within cranial cavity

malocclusion—abnormal position and contact of mandibular and maxillary teeth

microcephaly—abnormal smallness of the head

nystagmus—involuntary back-and-forth or up-and-down movements of the eye

papillae—small, rough elevations or projections

ENHANCED OUTLINE

I. Relevant health history

See text pages

A. Current status

    1. Does the client have frequent or severe headaches?

        a) Description (e.g., type, location, duration)

        b) Onset, frequency, and treatment

        c) Associated symptoms (e.g., nausea, visual disturbances)

    2. Does the client have any vision problems or eye pain?

    3. Does the client experience dizziness?

    4. Does the client experience frequent earaches or ringing in the ears?

    5. Does the client have any drainage from the ears?

        a) Description (e.g., appearance, odor)

        b) Frequency, onset, duration, and treatment

    6. Has the client noticed any recent changes in vision or hearing?

    7. Does the client have nasal discharge or postnasal drip?

    8. Does the client have nosebleeds?

        a) Onset, frequency, and duration

        b) Treatments

    9. Does the client take any medications, including over-the-counter (OTC) preparations? (See Nurse Alert, "Adverse Drug Reactions Affecting Head Structures.")

    10. Does the client have any allergies or sinus problems?

    11. Does the client have difficulty swallowing or frequent sore throats?

    12. What was the date of the client's last dental exam?

    13. Does the client have any chronic illnesses or health problems such as hypertension, diabetes, glaucoma, or thyroid dysfunction?

B. Past status

    1. Has the client ever had trauma to the head, face, or neck?

        a) Description

        b) Residual effects

    2. Has the client ever had surgery to any head or neck structure?

       a) Type and date of surgery

       b) Residual effects

    3. Has the client ever had a seizure?

       a) Type(s); type and date of last seizure

       b) Prescribed medication

       c) Any restrictions on daily activities

C. Family history

    1. Has anyone in the client's family been diagnosed with hearing or vision problems, including eye or ear diseases?

    2. Has anyone in the client's family had a history of seizures and if so, what type?

!   N U R S E   *A L E R T*   !

Adverse Drug Reactions Affecting Head Structures

Ask the client about current medications he/she is taking to assess adverse reactions, for example:

- Alopecia: may be caused by allopurinol, antilipemics, antineoplastics, or lithium salts
- Blurred vision: may be caused by aminoglycosides, antiarrhythmics, anticholinergics, non-steroidal anti-inflammatory drugs (NSAIDs), or genitourinary smooth muscle relaxants
- Photophobia: may be caused by anticholinergics, antiarrhythmics, or cardiotonic glycosides
- Tinnitus: may be caused by aminoglycosides, nonsteroidal anti-inflammatory drugs (NSAIDs), antimalarials, diuretics, nonnarcotic analgesics and antipyretics
- Epistaxis (nosebleed): may be caused by some antineoplastics, isotretinoin, or warfarin sodium
- Dry mouth: may be caused by amphetamines, anticholinergics, antidepressants, anti-hypertensives, nonsteroidal anti-inflammatory drugs (NSAIDs), cardiac medications, genitourinary smooth muscle relaxants, or lithium salts
- Mouth lesions: may be caused by antineoplastics, gold salts, nonsteroidal anti-inflammatory drugs (NSAIDs), or penicillamine
- Gingival hyperplasia: may be caused by phenytoin sodium

II. Anatomy and physiology

A. The head and neck
   1. Structure of the head
      a) Cranial bones (8): frontal, right and left parietal, right and left temporal, ethmoid, sphenoid, and occipital
      b) Face
         (1) Bones (14): vomer, mandible (movable), zygomatic (2), lacrimal, right and left maxillae, palatine (2), right and left nasal, and inferior nasal conchae (3)
         (2) Cranial nerve V (trigeminal nerve): transmits facial sensations; involved in chewing
         (3) Cranial nerve VII (facial nerve): innervates facial muscles; involved in taste
         (4) Temporal artery: major artery extending from in front of ear across temporal bone onto forehead
      c) Scalp

See text pages
_____

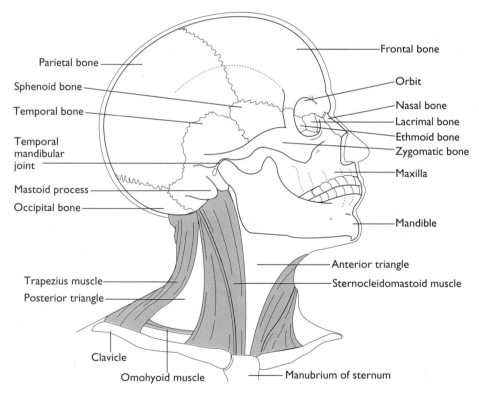

Figure 5–1
Structures of the Head and Neck

2. Structure of the neck: cervical vertebrae, ligaments and muscles, trachea, thyroid gland, cervical lymph nodes, and major vessels (carotid arteries and jugular veins)
    a) Major muscles: Trapezius and sternocleidomastoid provide neck support and allow movement.
    b) Anterior and posterior triangles
        (1) Anterior triangle: bounded by mandible, sternocleidomastoid muscles, and midline of trachea
        (2) Posterior triangle: bounded by sternocleidomastoid muscle, trapezius muscle, and clavicle

B. The eye
    1. External (extraocular) structures
        a) Eyelids (palpebrae): cover anterior eye, contain eyelashes, and protect and lubricate eye
        b) Conjunctivae: transparent membranes
            (1) Palpebral conjunctiva
                (a) Conjunctiva lines eyelids and appears shiny pink or red.
                (b) Meibomian glands appear as vertical yellow striations on inner lid margins and secrete sebum.
            (2) Bulbar conjunctiva: covers sclera, merging with corneal epithelium at limbus
        c) Lacrimal apparatus (lacrimal glands, puncta, lacrimal sac, and nasolacrimal duct)
            (1) Lacrimal gland is located superior and lateral to eye bulb; produces tears to lubricate cornea and conjunctivae.
            (2) Tears drain through puncta, openings in margin of upper and lower lids, and pass into lacrimal sac through the nasolacrimal duct and into the nose.
    2. Internal (intraocular) structures: The 3 layers of the eye are sclera, choroid, and retina.
        a) Sclera: outermost layer of eye; sensitive to touch
        b) Cornea: replaces sclera over pupil and iris
        c) Anterior and posterior chambers: contain aqueous humor
        d) Iris: diaphragm in front of lens; pigmented
        e) Pupil: opening at center of iris; constricts and dilates
        f) Lens: lies behind iris at pupillary opening; allows eye to focus
        g) Ciliary body: controls lens thickness and produces aqueous humor that drains through the canal of Schlemm
        h) Vitreous humor: gelatinous material; fills cavity behind lens
        i) Choroid: middle layer (beneath sclera) that contains numerous blood vessels; iris and ciliary body part of choroid

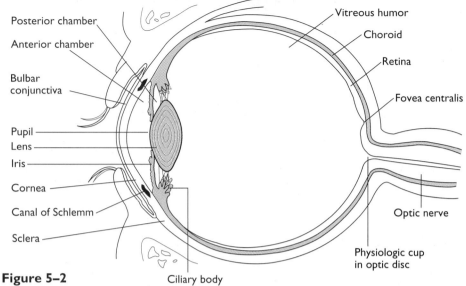

Figure 5–2
The Eye

Labels: Posterior chamber, Anterior chamber, Bulbar conjunctiva, Pupil, Lens, Iris, Cornea, Canal of Schlemm, Sclera, Ciliary body, Vitreous humor, Choroid, Retina, Fovea centralis, Optic nerve, Physiologic cup in optic disc

     j) Retina: innermost layer of eyeball that receives images and transmits impulses; contains rods and cones (visual receptors)
        (1) Nerve fibers exit retina and enter optic nerve (cranial nerve II) through optic disc (nasal side of retina); depression in temporal side of disc called physiologic cup.
        (2) Macula is lateral to optic disc on temporal side of retina; contains slight depression (fovea centralis retinae) with highest concentration of cones and most acute central vision.
        (3) Retinal vessels consist of 4 sets of arterioles and veins.
  3. Cranial nerves II, III, IV, V, VI, VII: innervate eye (see section II,B,1 of Chapter 12 for a discussion of cranial nerves)
  4. Rectus and oblique muscles: control eye movement

C. The ear
  1. External: auricle (pinna) and external auditory canal (meatus)
  2. Middle: small, air-filled cavity in temporal bone that is separated from external ear by tympanic membrane
    a) Tympanic membrane (eardrum)
        (1) This shiny, translucent membrane consists of layers of skin, fibrous tissue, and mucous membrane.
        (2) Handle of malleus attaches to inner surface of eardrum.
    b) Auditory ossicles
        (1) 3 small bones: malleus (hammer), incus (anvil), and stapes (stirrup)
        (2) Transmit sound
    c) 2 windows: oval window, into which stapes fits, and the membrane-covered round window, which opens to inner ear

   3. Eustachian tube: joins middle ear with nasopharynx; allows equalization of pressure between inner/outer surfaces of eardrum
   4. Inner ear: membranous labyrinth within body labyrinth, consisting of 3 parts (vestibule, semicircular canals, and cochlea)
      a) Vestibule and semicircular canals: involved in sensation of position and equilibrium
      b) Cochlea: coiled tube containing organ of Corti, which transmits sound to cochlear branch of auditory nerve

D. The nose
   1. Nasal cavity: divided into 2 halves by nasal septum; forms nostrils (nares) in external nose
   2. Path of air
      a) Enters through nostril (anterior naris)
      b) Passes into vestibule, where coarse hairs filter air
      c) Passes by inferior, middle, and superior turbinates
         (1) Turbinates are covered by highly vascular mucous membrane and protrude into nasal cavity laterally.
         (2) Below each turbinate is a cleft (meatus); each named for turbinate above (inferior, middle, and superior meatuses).
         (3) Area warms, filters, and humidifies air.
   3. Olfactory hair cells in roof of nasal cavity and upper third of septum: receptors for smell

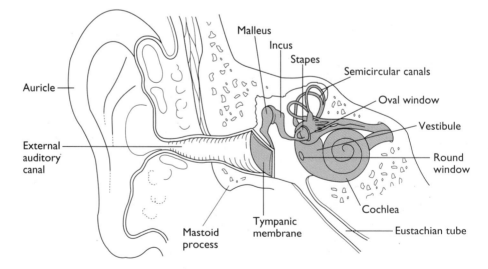

Figure 5–3
The Ear

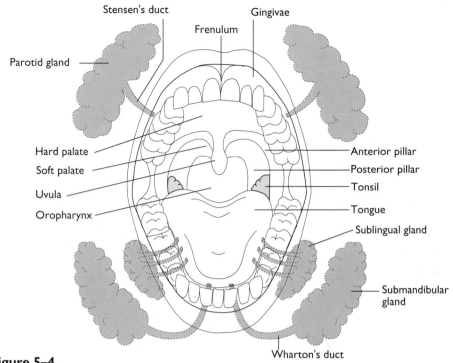

Figure 5–4
The Mouth and Oropharynx

4. Paranasal sinuses: air-filled cavities in bones of skull
    a) 4 sinuses: frontal, maxillary, sphenoidal, and ethmoidal
    b) Functions: aid in voice resonance; may also warm, moisten, and filter air

E. The mouth and oropharynx
    1. Mouth: bordered by lips anteriorly; contains tongue, gingivae, teeth, and salivary glands
        a) Tongue: covered with rough papillae and joined to mouth floor at midline by frenulum
        b) Gingivae (gums): mucous membrane and fibrous tissue attached to necks of teeth and alveolar margins of jaws
        c) Teeth: 32 adult, 16 in each jaw
        d) Salivary glands, 3 pairs: parotid, submandibular (submaxillary), and sublingual
            (1) Parotid: largest
                (a) Glands located just in front of and below auricles.
                (b) Parotid duct (Stensen's) opens into buccal mucosa near second upper molar.
            (2) Submandibular
                (a) Glands located below and in front of parotid glands.
                (b) Submandibular duct (Wharton's) opens on mouth floor on either side of frenulum.

(3) Sublingual (smallest): under tongue, opening onto mouth floor
  e) Hard and soft palates: Hard palate (anteriorly) and soft palate (posteriorly) separate roof of mouth and nasal cavity; uvula is suspended from middle of posterior edge of soft palate.
  2. Oropharynx: section of pharynx posterior to oral cavity; tonsils located on lateral walls

III. Assessment techniques

See text pages
_____

A. Approach: Be alert for signs of discomfort such as grimacing, stiffened posture, or holding of any part of head or neck during examination.

B. Inspection and palpation of the head
  1. Observe position of head (should be erect and still) as well as symmetry and size of skull (abnormalities include microcephaly and hydrocephaly).
  2. Part hair in several places to inspect scalp (remove hairpiece): Note hair distribution, texture, and quantity.
  3. Palpate head for symmetry and contour.
  4. Palpate scalp, using gentle rotary motion.
     a) Scalp should move freely over skull.
     b) Scalp should be free of lumps, depressions, lesions, scars, swelling, or tenderness.
     c) Hair should not be brittle or unusually dry or oily; however, be aware of cultural and individual grooming variations.

C. Inspection, palpation, and auscultation of the face
  1. Inspect face.
     a) Observe facial expressions; may reveal psychologic state, distress.
     b) Assess features for shape, symmetry, involuntary movement, or lack of movement.
     c) Assess skin color (pigmentation, pallor, cyanosis, jaundice) and texture; note any edema, lesions.
  2. Palpate skin.
     a) Palpation should reveal no pain or tenderness.
     b) Assess muscle function and tone: Have client smile, frown, puff out cheeks, show teeth while sides of face are palpated.
  3. Palpate and auscultate temporal arteries.
     a) Palpate pulses for equal strength and rhythm.
     b) Note any hardening or tenderness.
     c) Auscultate for bruits (blowing sounds) using stethoscope bell.
  4. Palpate temporomandibular joints (see section III,D,2 of Chapter 10).

D. Inspection, palpation, and auscultation of the neck
   1. Inspect neck for position, size, symmetry, masses, enlargement of glands or lymph nodes.
   2. Palpate anterior and posterior triangles.
      a) Note tenderness, masses; note muscle tone.
      b) Assess range of motion (ROM) including flexion (chin to chest), extension (head tilted backward), lateral rotation (side to side), lateral bending (ear to shoulder): Neck should be supple.
   3. Palpate lymph nodes: Palpate using fingertip pads in rotary motion; lymph nodes not normally palpable in healthy adults.
      a) Occipital: posterior at base of skull
      b) Postauricular: superficial over mastoid process
      c) Preauricular: in front of ear
      d) Tonsillar: at angle of mandible
      e) Submaxillary: halfway between angle and tip of mandible
      f) Submental: in midline behind tip of mandible
      g) Superficial cervical: anterior to sternocleidomastoid
      h) Posterior cervical: along anterior border of trapezius
      i) Deep cervical: deep to sternocleidomastoid; anterior to thyroid, larynx, trachea
      j) Supraclavicular: deep in angle formed by clavicle and sternocleidomastoid
   4. Palpate midline cartilages (thyroid cartilage, cricoid cartilage, and tracheal rings) and trachea: Palpate for symmetry and note any displacement or deviation.
   5. Inspect and palpate thyroid gland.
      a) Inspect for swelling or enlargement.
      b) Observe cartilage movement using tangential lighting.
         (1) Have client sip water with head tilted back slightly.
         (2) The thyroid gland, thyroid cartilage, and cricoid cartilage normally rise during swallowing (no unusual bulging should be seen).
      c) Palpate thyroid.
         (1) Palpate from behind, as client swallows.
         (2) Assess size, shape, consistency, presence of nodules.
   6. Inspect and palpate the cervical vertebrae: Assess for symmetry, tenderness, masses, or swelling.
   7. Inspect, palpate, and auscultate jugular veins and carotid arteries (see sections III,F and III,G of Chapter 7 for techniques).
      a) Note any jugular vein distention or visible arterial pulsations.
      b) Palpate for equal strength and rhythm; do not palpate both carotid arteries at the same time.
      c) Auscultate carotid arteries with stethoscope bell for bruits (client must hold breath).

E. Inspection and palpation of the eye
  1. Observe eye position and alignment.
  2. Inspect eyelids for ability to close, color, edema, scaling or lesions, and width and symmetry of palpebral fissures; inspect eyelashes for condition and position.
  3. Assess conjunctivae.
    a) Inspect bulbar conjunctivae.
      (1) Separate lids; ask client to look up, down, to each side.
      (2) Small blood vessels are normal.
    b) Inspect palpebral conjunctivae if client complains of eyelid pain or you suspect a foreign body.
      (1) Hold upper eyelashes and pull them gently downward; have client look down during this procedure.
      (2) Press on upper tarsal border with cotton-tipped applicator to evert eyelid (do not press on eye bulb).
      (3) Hold eyelashes to brow.
      (4) Palpebral conjunctivae should be pink with no foreign body or signs of swelling or infection.
      (5) Grasp upper eyelashes, pull gently forward, ask client to look up and blink: Lid should return to normal position.
  4. Assess lacrimal apparatus.
    a) Observe lacrimal gland and sac areas as well as puncta for signs of inflammation (e.g., redness, swelling, drainage).
    b) Press lacrimal sac inside lower inner orbital rim; fluid regurgitated through punctum indicates infection or nasolacrimal duct obstruction.
  5. Inspect sclera: normally white, but may have pigmented spots or be grayish blue in dark-skinned clients.
  6. Assess cornea, anterior chamber, and iris.
    a) Direct penlight from several side angles: Cornea and anterior chamber should be clear and transparent.
    b) Test for corneal reflex by gently touching wisp of cotton to cornea (both eyes should close when either is brushed).
    c) Observe iris shape and coloration (should appear flat, circular, symmetric).
  7. Assess pupils.
    a) Should be round and equal: Unequal pupil size (anisocoria) may indicate pathology.
    b) Assess response to light for direct and consensual reaction.
      (1) Darken room and direct penlight beam from the side to the anterior portion of 1 eye at a time.
      (2) Observe eye for direct response (constriction); observe other eye for consensual response.

c) Assess pupillary accommodation.
  (1) Ask client to stare at an object across the room (pupils will normally dilate).
  (2) Then ask client to fix gaze on object held approximately 5–6 inches from client's nose and brought toward bridge (both pupils should constrict and both eyes converge).
d) Document findings: PERRLA (pupils equally round, react to light, and accommodation).
8. Assess visual acuity.
  a) Use an eye chart, usually Snellen's eye chart (Snellen's E chart for preschool children or adults who cannot read).
    (1) Place client 20 feet away from chart in well-lit room.
    (2) Test 1 eye at a time, covering the other.
    (3) Record results for each eye and both eyes together; record whether corrective lens were worn.
    (4) Numerator is distance (20 feet) client is placed from chart; denominator is distance normal eye can read lettering.
  b) Refer clients with recording of 20/30 reading or greater to ophthalmologist.
  c) Assess near vision in clients over 40 years old.
9. Assess visual field (peripheral vision) if visual/neurologic defect is suspected: Gross confrontation test compares client's visual field with examiner's (if normal).
10. Assess extraocular muscles.
  a) 6 cardinal positions of gaze
    (1) Ask client to follow small object with eyes without moving head; move object through 6 cardinal positions.
    (2) Eyes should follow movement smoothly and symmetrically.
    (3) Watch for nystagmus, deviation of 1 eye, or inability to follow movement.
  b) Corneal light reflex test
    (1) Shine penlight between eyes from 12–15 inches away.
    (2) Asymmetrical reflections on corneas may indicate muscle weakness.
  c) Cover-uncover test: Assess both eyes separately.
    (1) Ask client to look at specific point with both eyes.
    (2) Cover 1 eye and observe other eye for attempt to fix on object.
    (3) Remove cover; jerky movement indicates muscle weakness (normally, eye movement should not be observed).
11. Perform ophthalmoscopic and tonometric examinations (advanced assessment techniques).
  a) Ophthalmoscopic assessment: Assesses internal structures.
  b) Tonometry: screening for glaucoma
    (1) Intraocular pressure is measured in all persons over 40 (over 30 if there is a family history of glaucoma).
    (2) Tonometry performed only by experienced examiners; uses Schiotz's tonometer.

F. Inspection and palpation of the ear
   1. External ear
      a) Inspect and palpate auricles.
         (1) Inspect for position, size, symmetry, or lesions.
         (2) Palpate for tenderness, swelling, or nodules.
         (3) Pull up auricle gently to assess for tenderness or pain.
      b) Examine behind ear for inflammation, nodules, or lesions; check ear for drainage.
   2. Internal ear (otoscopic examination)
      a) Use proper technique.
         (1) Tip client's head toward opposite shoulder.
         (2) Grasp auricle; pull upward and backward (down in infants and young children).
         (3) Insert speculum gently; change angle as needed.
      b) Inspect for discharge, inflammation, or foreign bodies.
      c) Assess cerumen.
         (1) Cerumen may vary in color and texture, but should be nearly odorless.
         (2) Remove by curettage or irrigation if view obstructed.
      d) Assess tympanic membrane.
         (1) Color: normally translucent and pearly gray; red, yellow, or white color may indicate disorder
         (2) Contour: should not bulge, be retracted or perforated
         (3) Landmarks
            (a) Light reflex: bright cone of light at 5 o'clock in right tympanic membrane and 7 o'clock in left
            (b) Long process, or handle of malleus: appears as whitish line from umbo to malleolar folds
            (c) Annulus: outer border, lighter in color
   3. Auditory function tests: Test 1 ear at a time, occluding other ear.
      a) Gross hearing tests
         (1) Whispered or spoken voice test: Whisper a word or phrase toward 1 ear from a distance of 1–2 feet away (be sure client cannot read your lips); client should repeat.
         (2) Ticking watch test: Move ticking watch away from client until client can no longer hear sound (first determine average distance at which ticking of your watch is heard by several persons with normal hearing).
      b) Weber test: tests lateralization of hearing
         (1) Strike tuning fork and place in middle of forehead or in middle top anterior portion of skull.
         (2) Ask client if he/she hears sound better in 1 ear or the other (client should hear sound equally in both ears).

    c) Rinne test: compares bone and air conduction
      (1) Place base of vibrating tuning fork on mastoid process.
      (2) When client can no longer hear sound, immediately place vibrating head of tuning fork ½–1 inch from meatus.
      (3) Sound normally heard twice as long through air than through bone
        (a) Heard longer in bone: conductive hearing loss
        (b) Heard longer in air but not twice as long as in bone: sensorineural hearing loss

G. Inspection and palpation of the nose
  1. External nose
    a) Inspect for symmetry and contour and for nasal flaring.
    b) Palpate for pain, tenderness, swelling, or deformity.
    c) Assess nasal patency: Press 1 naris at a time and have client breathe in through opposite naris.
    d) Press gently on tip of nose and shine penlight into nares: Inspect for tenderness, asymmetry, or deformity.
  2. Internal nose: Use otoscope with short, wide nasal speculum or nasal speculum with penlight.
    a) Lift tip of nose, insert closed speculum, open it slowly.
    b) Inspect mucosa.
      (1) Mucosa should be moist pink to red with no drainage, edema, inflammation, lesions, or polyps.
      (2) Describe any exudate (e.g., watery, purulent, bloody).
    c) Inspect septum for deviation, inflammation, or perforation (some deviation is normal).
    d) Inspect inferior and middle turbinates by tipping client's head back and inspecting for exudate, polyps, swelling: Describe any exudate.

H. Palpation, percussion, and transillumination of frontal and maxillary sinuses
  1. Palpate sinuses: Tenderness or pain may indicate sinusitis.
    a) Frontal sinuses: Press upward gently from under the bony ridge of upper orbit on each side.
    b) Maxillary sinuses: Press up gently on each side of face below zygomatic bone (cheekbone).
  2. Percuss sinus: Pain may indicate sinusitis.
    a) Frontal sinuses: Lightly tap just above eyebrows with index finger.
    b) Maxillary sinuses: Gently tap index or middle finger beneath eye in line with pupil.
  3. Transilluminate in darkened room if sinusitis is suspected: Reddish glow is normal; absence of glow indicates congestion or lack of sinus development.
    a) Frontal sinuses: Place light source against medial aspect of each supraorbital rim; look for dim red glow as light is transmitted just above eyebrow.
    b) Maxillary sinuses: Place light source lateral to nose, just beneath medial aspect of eye; look through client's open mouth for illumination of hard palate.

I. Inspection and palpation of the mouth
   1. Examination of the mouth and oropharynx
      a) Inspect lips for color, symmetry, inflammation, and lesions.
      b) Examine mouth with tongue blade and good light, noting any mouth odors throughout examination.
         (1) Oral mucosal surfaces: moist and light pink (patchy brown or bluish in dark-skinned clients) with no lesions or edema
         (2) Gums pink and firm: Inspect for inflammation, swelling, bleeding.
         (3) Teeth: Inspect for caries, missing teeth, malocclusions, and discolorations.
         (4) Tongue
            (a) Inspect dorsum for color, size, and any lesions: Whitish film normally covers tongue, papillae protrude.
            (b) Inspect lateral areas and undersurface of tongue.
               i) Ask client to move tongue from side to side and protrude it; inspect for symmetry.
               ii) With gloved hand, grasp tip of tongue with gauze and pull to left and then to right; note whitish or reddened patches, nodules, ulcers.
               iii) Palpate for induration or any lesions.
               iv) Ask client to touch tip of tongue to palate to inspect undersurface.
         (5) Frenulum, submandibular glands, and sublingual fold: Inspect during assessment of undersurface of tongue.
         (6) Hard and soft palates
            (a) Hard palate is lighter and rougher; soft palate is normally pink.
            (b) Inspect and palpate for any lesions, tenderness, swelling, deformities.
      c) Oropharynx: Examine size of uvula and tonsils.
         (1) Ask client to say "Ah" while placing tongue depressor on tongue to observe rise of uvula and soft palate.
         (2) Uvula should be midline; soft palate and uvula should rise symmetrically.
   2. Evaluation of gag reflex (performed only when there are signs of dysfunction)
      a) Press on posterior tongue with tongue blade.
      b) Decreased or absent gag reflex may indicate glossopharyngeal or vagus nerve dysfunction.

IV. Essential nursing care for client with neck pain

See text pages
_____

A. Nursing assessment
1. Gather relevant health history information (same as section I of this chapter).
2. Palpate the neck and assess range of motion; note muscle spasms, tenderness, or pain.
3. Assess the level of stress the client is experiencing.

B. Nursing diagnoses
1. High risk for altered health maintenance related to knowledge deficit concerning relationship between occupational stress and neck pain
2. High risk for altered health maintenance related to knowledge deficit concerning normal neck physiology
3. Alteration in comfort related to muscle tenseness
4. Impaired physical mobility related to neck pain

C. Nursing implementation (intervention)
1. Explain relationship between tension and neck pain to client.
2. Educate client regarding neck physiology and physiologic causes of neck pain.
3. Instruct client concerning methods of pain relief, including analgesics, application of warm compresses, relaxation techniques, and stress reduction methods.

D. Nursing evaluation
1. Client demonstrates through verbalization an understanding of neck physiology and the possible causes of neck pain.
2. Client takes positive steps to relieve work-related stress.
3. Client appropriately uses methods for pain relief.
4. Client experiences improved mobility and reduced pain.

1. Which of the following is important to remember when assessing a client's head?

   a. The size and shape of the cranium
   should be approximately the same in all
   clients of the same chronologic age.

   b. The cranium should contain identical
   structures in all clients of the same
   chronologic age.

   c. Palpation of a normal cranium will reveal no irregularities.

   d. Percussion and auscultation are particularly useful when assessing the cranium.

2. A 35-year-old female client reports that she
has been experiencing headaches recently.
She describes the headaches as a tight sensation in her temporal areas, lasting 3–6
hours, and occurring about 3 times per
week. She also states that she has noticed
some sensitivity to light when she has a
headache. Which of the following would be
the best response for the nurse to make?

   a. "Headaches are almost always of no con-
   sequence in people of your age. I don't
   think you have anything to worry about."

   b. "Have any other members of your family
   experienced frequent headaches? Sometimes there is a genetic link."

   c. "Can you tell me what you do to relieve the
   headaches? Have you tried any of the over-
   the-counter analgesics for pain?"

   d. "Frequent headaches are always a cause
   for concern. I will refer you to a specialist
   for a complete workup."

3. The nurse asks a 40-year-old client who has
come in for an eye examination if he uses
any OTC or prescription medications. The
client seems surprised by this question and
asks why this information is important.
Which of the following would be the best response for the nurse to make?

   a. "Some medications produce adverse reactions that can affect the structures of the
   head, including the eyes."

   b. "It is important for me to know if you
   need any additional prescriptions or
   refills."

   c. "We always take a medication history so
   we can make sure you are taking the correct amount of medication."

   d. "We always take a medication history so
   we can identify clients who may be abus-
   ing drugs."

4. Testing range of motion (ROM) in a client's
neck helps the nurse assess which of the following most directly?

   a. The presence of swollen lymph nodes or
   masses

   b. Muscle and joint function

   c. Swelling of the cervical vertebrae

   d. Thyroid gland enlargement

5. A 78-year-old client has come for a periodic
eye exam. Which of the following would be a
normal finding in this client?

   a. A visual acuity of 20/200

   b. Hardness of the eyeball noticeable on
   palpation

   c. Exotropia, in which the axis of 1 eye
   turns outward

   d. An opaque, gray to white ring surrounding the cornea

6. A 42-year-old female client complains of eye
pain. Inspection and palpation of the eye reveal a very tender, pimplelike lesion at the
border of the lower eyelid, pointing on the
lid margin. These assessment findings lead
most clearly to a:

   a. Xanthelasma.

   b. Hordeolum.

   c. Lacrimal sac inflammation.

   d. Chalazion.

7. A nurse is examining the ears of a 2-month-
old male infant. The nurse finds that the
top of the infant's auricles are at a level below the lateral angle of the eye. Which of

the following would be the most appropriate nursing action?

a. The nurse should perform further assessment of the infant because low-set ears suggest chromosomal or renal abnormalities.

b. The nurse should perform further assessment of the infant's eyes because such a position may indicate problems with internal eye structures.

c. A detailed auditory assessment is indicated since low-set ears indicate a problem with hearing.

d. No further assessment of the infant is needed because ears in this position are a familial trait.

8. A woman has brought her 17-month-old son to the clinic. She tells the nurse that he doesn't make many sounds and relies on gestures to get what he wants. She states that her older children were able to talk at this age. She is concerned that he may have hearing loss. Which of the following questions would best help the nurse investigate this problem?

a. "Have you noticed your son pulling at either of his ears?"

b. "Does your son respond to loud or unusual noises?"

c. "Have you noticed any problem with his coordination or balance?"

d. "Is your son taking any OTC nasal decongestants?"

9. Which of the following is true about the physical assessment of an adult's ear?

a. Periodic hearing screening is not necessary because an adult can report if he/she is experiencing hearing loss.

b. Inspection of the outer ear is sufficient unless the client is experiencing ear pain.

c. Palpation of the outer structure of the ear yields no useful results.

d. The middle and inner ear cannot be inspected, so the nurse must assess their function through hearing testing.

10. The nurse is examining the nose and sinuses of an 18-year-old client. The client has been involved in a motor vehicle accident in which his forehead struck the steering wheel. The nurse finds that the client's nasal septum is deviated and he has clear, thin nasal secretions. The client reports that he is just getting over a cold. Which of the following is the best nursing action for this client?

a. The nurse should further assess the nasal drainage.

b. The nurse should tell the client to apply cold compresses to the forehead and nose for 10 minutes at a time.

c. No nursing action is indicated.

d. The nurse should assess the client's abdomen and extremities for other injuries.

11. Which of the following should the nurse keep in mind when assessing the head and neck of a pediatric client?

a. The assessment of a pediatric client does not differ from that of an adult.

b. Children under age 5 are not able to follow directions sufficiently to have their hearing tested.

c. All children age 2 and under should have their head circumference measured.

d. Visual acuity cannot be assessed in children until they are able to read.

12. Which of the following should the nurse keep in mind when assessing the head and neck of an elderly client?

a. The assessment of an elderly client does not differ from that of other clients.

b. Decreases in visual acuity should be expected in all clients at age 50.

c. Elderly clients experience memory loss and cannot be considered reliable historians.

d. Elderly clients may experience decreased range of motion (ROM) as a part of aging.

1. Correct answer is b. While it is true that the size and shape of the cranium vary from person to person, the structures of the cranium do not vary.

a. The size and shape of the cranium vary greatly in individuals of the same chronologic age.
c. Palpation will reveal irregularities in a normal skull, especially near the suture lines between the parietal and occipital bones. No lesions or marked asymmetry should be present, however.
d. Percussion and auscultation are not useful tools for assessing the cranium. Inspection and palpation are the primary means of assessment.

2. Correct answer is c. Her symptoms are descriptive of a muscle contraction headache, although further information is needed by the nurse. A report about whether pain is relieved by an OTC analgesic would provide further data.

a. This response minimizes the client's concern. The nurse does not have sufficient data to make this decision.
b. Headaches have not been proven to have a familial link. This is false information.
d. The nurse does not have enough information to refer the client for a more extensive examination. Such a response may alarm the client unnecessarily.

3. Correct answer is a. Adverse reactions that affect the eye, such as blurred vision and visual disturbances, are among the most commonly reported.

b. It is not necessary for the nurse to be concerned at this point about the client's need to have medications prescribed or refilled.
c. Although this may be a secondary reason for taking a medication history, it is not the primary reason in this case.

d. Although the nurse should keep this in mind when assessing all clients, this is not the primary reason for completing a medication history.

4. Correct answer is b. Testing ROM in the neck helps the nurse assess how the client's muscles and joints are functioning. Normally the client can move the neck a certain distance in degrees in a number of different directions.

a. Inspection and palpation would help the nurse assess the presence of swollen lymph nodes or masses.
c. Inspection and palpation would help the nurse assess swelling of the cervical vertebrae.
d. Inspection and palpation of the neck would help the nurse assess thyroid gland enlargement.

5. Correct answer is d. Called arcus senilis, this condition is normal in the elderly and is caused by lipid deposits. It does not interfere with vision.

a. A visual acuity of 20/200 would be normal only in an infant.
b. Hardness of the eyeball that can be felt on palpation may indicate increased intraocular pressure such as that caused by glaucoma, an abnormal condition. Further assessment would be necessary through tonometry.
c. Exotropia is caused by severe ocular muscle weakness. It is an abnormal condition in any age group.

6. Correct answer is b. A hordeolum is an infection of 1 of the meibomian glands of the eyelid and appears as a painful, pimplelike red lesion that points on the lid margin.

a. A xanthelasma appears as 1 or a group of raised, yellow plaques at the nasal portion of 1 or both eyelids.
c. An inflammation of the lacrimal sac appears as a swelling between the lower eyelid and nose.
d. A chalazion is also an inflammation of 1 of the meibomian glands but is usually painless and generally points inside the lid rather than on the margin.

7. **Correct answer is a.** Low-set ears are often an indicator of renal and chromosomal abnormalities. Such ear placement always requires further assessment.

b. Placement of the eyes in relation to the ears is not an indicator of any abnormalities of the internal eye structures.
c. Low-set ears may indicate other types of problems, but not problems with auditory function.
d. While the size and shape of the ears may reflect familial traits, the position of the ears does not.

8. **Correct answer is b.** Lack of response to loud or unusual noises is a good indicator of hearing loss. If the parent responds negatively, referral to a hearing specialist is indicated.

a and **c.** Both of these questions would help the nurse assess whether the child had an ear infection. Many children who are experiencing ear pain from ear infections tug at their ears; ear infections can also cause problems with equilibrium.
d. This question would not help the nurse assess possible hearing loss. Although some OTC medications can cause adverse reactions involving the ears, decongestants are not included in this category.

9. **Correct answer is d.** Assessment of the middle and inner ear must occur through the indirect method of hearing testing. These structures cannot be adequately observed in a noninvasive manner.

a. The client is often the last person to recognize his/her own hearing loss.
b. A complete ear exam includes more than just inspection of the outer ear. A number of ear disorders do not cause pain.
c. Palpation of the external ear is a useful part of the assessment.

10. **Correct answer is a.** Given the nature of the injuries, this may be cerebrospinal fluid leaking from a basal skull fracture. Clear nasal secretions are not typical for a client who is getting over a cold; secretions are usually thick and may be green or yellow. This client may have a very serious injury and needs further assessment promptly. Examining the drainage is a logical first step.

b. This would be appropriate if the nurse suspected minor injury to the soft tissues of the face. Bruising and localized swelling, not thin nasal secretions, would be consistent with such injuries.
c. The client clearly needs further assessment because of the potential seriousness of these injuries.
d. Although the client does need further assessment, the priority nursing action should be to investigate the source of the nasal secretions.

11. **Correct answer is c.** The brain grows very rapidly in the first 2 years, making measurements of head circumference an important assessment tool. The anterior fontanel closes at about 18 months and the posterior fontanel at 2 months. Head circumference increases by only about 2 cm during the toddler years.

a. A number of findings are different between children and adults and the 2 groups therefore require different assessment procedures.
b. This is not true. Children under age 5 are able to understand and follow simple instructions.
d. Visual acuity in children who cannot read can be assessed with pictures of common objects.

12. **Correct answer is d.** A decrease in normal ROM is a common finding in elderly clients.

a. The elderly client does differ from adults of other ages; for example, visual and auditory acuity diminishes.
b. Decreased visual acuity in elderly clients does occur but it cannot be expected in all clients; besides, age 50 is not elderly.
c. Elderly clients can be very reliable historians. Memory loss is not a normal finding.

6

The Respiratory System

OVERVIEW

I. Relevant health history
  A. Current status
  B. Past status
  C. Family history

II. Anatomy and physiology
  A. Thorax
  B. Upper airways
  C. Lungs

III. Assessment techniques
  A. Approach
  B. Inspection of the thorax
  C. Palpation of the thorax and trachea

  D. Percussion of the thorax
  E. Auscultation of the lungs
  F. Diagnostic tests

IV. Essential nursing care for client with suspected asthma
  A. Nursing assessment
  B. Nursing diagnoses
  C. Nursing implementation (intervention)
  D. Nursing evaluation

NURSING HIGHLIGHTS

1. The nurse should be aware that respiratory system changes will alter other body systems and that changes in other body systems may affect the respiratory system.
2. Lung disease is the third leading cause of death in the United States, and cigarette smoking is the leading cause of lung cancer, emphysema, and chronic bronchitis.
3. Lung disease is often preventable: The nurse should educate the client about avoiding respiratory hazards, especially cigarette smoke (see Client Teaching Checklist, "Preventing Lung Disease").
4. The nurse should keep in mind that the very young, the elderly, and those with compromised immune systems, such as clients with AIDS, are at greatest risk for acute respiratory infections.

GLOSSARY

bifurcate—to divide into 2 parts or branches
costal margin—lower edge of rib cage near xiphoid process
diffusion—movement of molecules across membranes from an area of higher
   concentration to an area of lower concentration
fremitus—palpable vibrations, especially of the chest wall
polycythemia—an abnormal increase in the concentration of red blood cells;
   sometimes related to pulmonary or heart disease
pulmonary perfusion—gas exchange in alveoli
serous membrane—thin membrane that secretes a watery fluid

ENHANCED OUTLINE

I. Relevant health history

A. Current status (see Client Teaching Checklist, "Warning Signs of Lung
   Disease")

> See text pages
> _____

See text pages

   1. Does the client have a cough?
      a) Description (e.g., moist or dry, barking or hacking)
      b) Time of occurrence

2. Does the client produce sputum with the cough?
   a) Description
      (1) Color
         (a) Clear to white: not infected
         (b) Yellow or green sputum: a sign of infection or disease (e.g., tuberculosis)
         (c) Rust-colored or blood-streaked sputum: may indicate pulmonary edema, pneumonia, or tuberculosis
      (2) Amount (e.g., scant, copious) and consistency (thin, thick, frothy, viscid [sticky], mucopurulent)
      (3) Odor: odorless or with fetid (foul) odor
   b) When and how often sputum is produced (e.g., sputum originating from draining sinuses may result in a productive cough)
3. Does the client experience shortness of breath?
   a) Time of occurrence
      (1) With activity: may indicate a breathing disorder or other health alteration (e.g., disease, obesity)
      (2) During sleep, awakening client: may indicate lung disease or cardiac dysfunction
   b) Frequency
   c) Associated symptoms (e.g., chest pain, heart palpitations)
4. Does the client smoke? If so, how much and for how long has he/she been smoking?
5. Does the client have allergies?
   a) Identification of allergens (e.g., pollens, foods, animal dander)
   b) Description of symptoms
   c) Treatments
6. Does the client have a chronic disease such as cardiovascular disease?
7. Is the client exposed to environmental irritants?
   a) Potential irritants include cigarette smoke, paint, sprays, dust, pollution, coal dust, asbestos fibers, grain dust, and fertilizers.
   b) Educate the client about how to avoid exposure (see Client Teaching Checklist, "Avoiding Respiratory Irritants and Carcinogens").
8. Does the client live in crowded conditions, increasing exposure to infection?

B. Past status
   1. Has the client ever been exposed to respiratory irritants?
      a) Identification of irritant
      b) Duration of exposure (estimated)
   2. Has the client ever had a breathing problem or respiratory illness?
      a) Description of problem, including cause and symptoms
      b) Treatments

Avoiding Respiratory Irritants and Carcinogens

Instruct the client to recognize and avoid the following respiratory irritants:

✔ Tobacco smoke
✔ Radon
✔ Asbestos
✔ Dust (textile, coal, lead, grain)
✔ Silica
✔ Household chemicals, fertilizers
✔ Allergens (pollen, molds, dust mites)
✔ Outdoor air pollution

C. Family history
　　1. Has anyone in the client's family been diagnosed with emphysema, allergies, tuberculosis, or lung cancer?
　　2. Does anyone in the client's family smoke, exposing others to secondhand smoke?

II. Anatomy and physiology

A. Thorax

See text pages
_____

　　1. Skeletal components
　　　　a) Sternum
　　　　　　(1) Manubrium
　　　　　　(2) Body
　　　　　　(3) Xiphoid process
　　　　b) Ribs: 12 pairs
　　　　　　(1) Posterior attachment to vertebral column
　　　　　　(2) Anterior attachment to sternum or costal cartilage of rib above
　　　　　　(3) 2 lowest ribs (11th and 12th): not attached to any part of thorax anteriorly (floating ribs)
　　　　　　(4) Spaces between ribs: intercostal spaces
　　　　c) Thoracic vertebrae: 12
　　2. Thoracic cavities
　　　　a) Pleural cavities
　　　　　　(1) Right pleural cavity: contains right lung
　　　　　　(2) Left pleural cavity: contains left lung
　　　　　　(3) Pleura: serous membrane lining pleural cavities
　　　　　　　　(a) Parietal pleural membrane: lines the chest wall and diaphragm
　　　　　　　　(b) Visceral pleural membrane: lines the outside of the lung
　　　　　　(4) Pleural space: potential space between the parietal and visceral pleural membranes

      b) Mediastinum

        (1) Separates pleural cavities

        (2) Contains organs such as the heart, large blood vessels, trachea, and esophagus

  3. Functions of the thorax

    a) Supports lungs

    b) Protects lungs

    c) Allows for lung expansion and contraction

    d) Protects mediastinal organs

  4. Landmarks of the thorax: The nurse should remember to refer to thoracic landmarks when describing the location of findings.

    a) Suprasternal notch: depression above anterior thorax

    b) Angle of Louis, or manubriosternal junction

      (1) Visible, palpable articulation between manubrium and sternum body where second rib joins sternum

      (2) Helpful in locating and identifying ribs

    c) Ribs (see section II,A,1,b of this chapter)

    d) Costal angle: angle formed by the lower borders of the ribs (costal margin) where they intersect with the sternum

    e) Midsternal line: runs vertically through the middle of the sternum

    f) Midclavicular lines: run vertically through the middle of the clavicles

    g) Anterior axillary lines: run vertically through anterior axillary folds

    h) Posterior axillary lines: run vertically through posterior axillary folds

    i) Midaxillary lines: run vertically through the center of the axillae between anterior and posterior axillary lines

    j) Vertebra prominens

      (1) Prominent spinous process at C7 (seventh cervical vertebra)

      (2) Palpable and most prominent when neck is flexed anteriorly: When two processes appear equally prominent, superior one is process at C7 and inferior one is process at T1.

    k) Midspinal line: runs vertically along posterior vertebrae

    l) Scapular lines: run vertically through the inferior angles of the scapulae

    m) Scapulae

    n) Clavicles

5. Thoracic structures
   a) Trachea: bifurcates at the Angle of Louis anteriorly and T4 posteriorly
   b) Lungs
      (1) The apex of each lung is 2–4 cm above inner third of clavicle anteriorly.
      (2) Lower border of lung is at approximately T10 (may extend to T12 with deep inspiration) posteriorly, the sixth rib at midclavicular line, and the eighth rib at midaxillary line.
   c) Esophagus, heart, and great blood vessels: located in the mediastinum
   d) Diaphragm: borders on expiration
      (1) Anterior borders
         (a) Right dome at fifth rib, midclavicular line
         (b) Left dome at sixth rib
      (2) Posterior border: at T10
      (3) Lateral border: at eighth rib, midaxillary line
6. Inspiration and expiration: movement of thoracic cage
   a) Inspiration
      (1) Diaphragm descends and flattens.
      (2) Intercostal muscles contract.
      (3) Lungs expand.
      (4) Ribs flare.
   b) Expiration
      (1) Diaphragm rises.
      (2) Intercostal muscles relax.
      (3) Lungs expel air.

B. Upper airways
   1. Structures: mouth, nose, pharynx, larynx, trachea
   2. Functions
      a) Act as air passageways
      b) Filter, warm, and moisten air

C. Lungs: paired, asymmetric
   1. Structures
      a) Bronchi
         (1) Bronchi branch right and left from the trachea; divide further into 5 branches within each lung.
         (2) Right bronchus is more vertical, shorter, wider than left.
      b) Bronchioles
         (1) Arise from the bronchi
         (2) Lead to alveolar sacs
      c) Alveolar sacs
         (1) End in alveoli
         (2) Exchange oxygen and carbon dioxide
      d) Pleura (see section II,A,2,a of this chapter)

    e) Fissures

        (1) Both lungs are divided into upper and lower lobes by oblique fissures from T3 to the sixth rib at the midclavicular line.

        (2) Right lung is divided into a third (middle) lobe by horizontal fissure proceeding from the right midaxillary line at the fifth rib posteriorly to the fourth rib anteriorly.

2. Functions

    a) Gas exchange: occurs through ventilation, pulmonary perfusion, and diffusion

    b) Protection: Mucus catches foreign particles, cilia remove them.

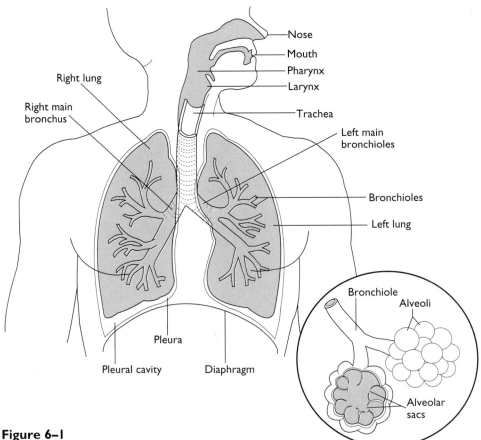

Figure 6–1
The Respiratory System

III. Assessment techniques

See text pages
_____

A. Approach
   1. Client should be undressed to waist, covered with a gown.
   2. Lighting should be adequate.
   3. Client should be sitting (supine if client cannot sit).
   4. Room should be warm.

B. Inspection of the thorax
   1. Configuration
      a) Normal findings
         (1) Chest expands equally and symmetrically.
         (2) Costal angle is <90°.
         (3) Anteroposterior diameter is less than transverse diameter by ratio of approximately 1:2–5:7.
         (4) Ribs are attached to vertebral column at 45° angle.
      b) Developmental variations (see sections II,B and III,B of Chapter 3)
      c) Abnormal findings
         (1) Retractions: depression of chest soft tissues on inspiration (usually in intercostal spaces; may also appear in supraclavicular and infraclavicular regions)
         (2) Barrel chest
            (a) Condition in which the anteroposterior diameter of the thorax is increased in relation to the transverse diameter; ratio is nearly 1:1.
            (b) Normal in infancy; often seen in older adults
         (3) Pectus excavatum (funnel chest): abnormal depression of the lower sternum creating a funnel shape; ribs horizontal
         (4) Pectus carinatum (pigeon breast): abnormal anterior sternal protrusion
         (5) Spinal abnormalities
            (a) Lordosis: anterior spinal curvature
            (b) Scoliosis: lateral spinal curvature
            (c) Kyphosis: exaggerated rounding of thoracic spine
            (d) Kyphoscoliosis: lateral curvature of the spine accompanying rounded thoracic hump
         (6) Flail chest: segment of unattached (fractured) ribs resulting in paradoxical movement of that area inward during inspiration and outward during expiration
         (7) Chest wall bulging
   2. Assessment of respiratory effort
      a) Skin color
         (1) Normal findings (see section III,B,1 of Chapter 4)
         (2) Abnormal findings
            (a) Blue coloring may be a sign of decreased oxygen in the blood, or cyanosis.

  (b) Ruddy complexion may be normal or the result of polycythemia.

 b) Fingers: Clubbing (see section III,D,2,b of Chapter 4) may indicate chronic pulmonary or cardiovascular disease.

 c) Respiratory pattern

  (1) Normal findings

   (a) Regular rhythm

   (b) Quiet and unlabored

   (c) Adult rate: 14–20 breaths/minute

   (d) Infant, pediatric, and gerontologic rates: See sections II,B; III,B; and IV,B of Chapter 3.

  (2) Abnormal findings

   (a) Hyperpnea: rapid or deep breathing (may occur with pain, disease, drugs, hysteria, high altitude, or normally with exercise)

   (b) Tachypnea: rapid breathing (may occur with pleuritic chest pain, fractured rib, or hysteria)

   (c) Bradypnea: slow breathing (may occur with diabetic coma, drug-induced respiratory depression, or central nervous system disturbance)

   (d) Obstructive breathing: prolonged expiration and air trapping (may occur with lung disease)

   (e) Hyperventilation: increase in breathing rate and depth resulting in excessive intake of oxygen and loss of carbon dioxide (may occur with anxiety or metabolic acidosis)

   (f) Cheyne-Stokes respiration: periods of apnea and hyperpnea (may occur with cerebral hemorrhage or heart failure)

   (g) Biot's breathing: irregular breathing with periods of apnea (may occur with central nervous system disorders; sometimes occurs normally)

   (h) Kussmaul's respiration: abnormally rapid but deep breathing (may occur with renal disease or diabetic acidosis)

   (i) Hypopnea: decreased breathing rate and depth (may occur with pain or may occur normally in athletes)

   (j) Hypoventilation: decreased breathing rate and depth resulting in decreased levels of oxygen, increased carbon dioxide, or both (may occur with bronchitis or emphysema)

   (k) Apnea: breathing temporarily stops (may occur with heart disease or brain injury)

d) Breathing methods
    (1) Thoracic breathing
        (a) Upward and outward motion of chest
        (b) Common in adult females
    (2) Abdominal breathing
        (a) Breathing with abdominal muscles
        (b) Common during sleep
        (c) Common in infants and adult males
    (3) Purse-lipped breathing: common in clients with chronic obstructive pulmonary disease (COPD)
    (4) Use of accessory neck muscles to breathe: sign of respiratory distress
    (5) Nasal flaring: sign of respiratory distress

C. Palpation of the thorax and trachea
  1. Assessment of trachea position
    a) Procedure
      (1) Place thumb on each side of trachea above suprasternal notch.
      (2) Move thumbs along clavicles to sternocleidomastoid muscles.
    b) Normal findings: Distance to each sternocleidomastoid muscle should be equal, indicating a midline trachea.
    c) Abnormal findings: Lateral deviation may indicate a disease or disorder.
  2. General assessment of the thorax
    a) Procedure
      (1) Palpate with fingertips and palms of 1 or both hands.
      (2) Move systematically from 1 area to the next and compare corresponding areas.
        (a) Anterior thorax: Proceed from supraclavicular to infraclavicular, sternal, xiphoid, rib, and axillary areas.
        (b) Posterior thorax: Proceed from supraclavicular to interscapular, infrascapular, and lateral walls of thorax.
    b) Normal findings
      (1) Skin is warm, smooth, and dry.
      (2) Areas are symmetrical.
      (3) Aortic pulsations are normal and regular.
    c) Abnormal findings
      (1) Skin lesions
      (2) Tenderness or pain
      (3) Abnormal pulsations
      (4) Bulges
      (5) Masses
      (6) Abnormal movements
      (7) Crepitus
      (8) Asymmetry

3. Assessment of respiratory excursion
   a) Procedure
      (1) Anterior thorax
         (a) Place hands on the chest wall.
         (b) Position thumbs along costal margin an equal distance from the sternum in the intercostal spaces below the fifth or sixth intercostal space.
         (c) Observe client during a deep inspiration.
      (2) Posterior thorax
         (a) Place thumbs at level of tenth rib on both sides of spine with palms on posterolateral chest wall.
         (b) Observe client during a deep inspiration.
   b) Normal finding: Thumbs should move apart equally.
   c) Abnormal findings
      (1) Asymmetrical expansion
      (2) Decreased range of expansion
4. Assessment of fremitus
   a) Procedure
      (1) Use the palmar aspects of the fingers, the ball of the hand, the ulnar aspect of the hand, or a closed fist.
      (2) Place hands on corresponding sides of the chest wall (or if using 1 hand, move from 1 side to the corresponding side of the chest).
      (3) Have client repeat words such as "ninety-nine," or "one, two, three."
      (4) Compare vibrations of each lung.
   b) Normal findings
      (1) Moderate vibrations
      (2) Most intense in first and second intercostal spaces near bronchial bifurcation
   c) Abnormal findings
      (1) Decreased or absent fremitus: may indicate bronchial obstruction, pneumothorax, or COPD
      (2) Increased fremitus: may indicate pneumonia, pulmonary fibrosis, or a lung tumor
      (3) Pleural friction rub (grating vibration): may indicate pneumonia, tuberculosis, pleurisy, or pulmonary embolism

D. Percussion of the thorax
   1. Purposes: to determine lung boundaries and to determine relative amounts of liquid, air, or solids in lung

2. Procedure
    a) Use mediate (indirect) percussion: finger of 1 hand (pleximeter) held against area to be assessed and struck with finger of other hand (plexor).
        (1) Press middle finger of nondominant hand firmly on area to be percussed; keep other fingers and palm off skin surface.
        (2) Tap distal joint of pleximeter once or twice with plexor (usually middle finger of dominant hand).
        (3) Keep wrist of striking hand loosely flexed; use quick, snapping motion.
        (4) Remove plexor as soon as blow is delivered.
    b) Percuss anterior, lateral, and posterior chest wall.
    c) Percuss over intercostal spaces, not bones.
    d) Note percussion sounds.
        (1) Intensity
        (2) Pitch
        (3) Duration
        (4) Quality
    e) Compare sounds on corresponding sides.
    f) Percuss according to set sequence.
        (1) Anterior
            (a) Percuss lung apices in supraclavicular area.
            (b) Move downward from side to side 3–5 cm at a time.
            (c) Normal sounds are resonant from below clavicle to the fifth intercostal space (right side) and to the third intercostal space (left side).
        (2) Lateral: Position client's arm above head.
            (a) Begin at axilla.
            (b) Percuss intercostal spaces.
            (c) Normal sounds are resonant to the sixth or eighth intercostal space.
        (3) Posterior
            (a) Begin in the suprascapular area.
            (b) Move from left to right at 3–5 cm intervals to interscapular and infrascapular areas.
            (c) Normal sounds are resonant to level of T10.
3. Normal findings
    a) Resonance (hollow, loud, low pitch, long duration): heard over adult lung
    b) Hyperresonance (booming, very loud, very low pitch, very long duration): heard over a child's lung and sometimes in very thin adults
    c) Dullness (thudlike, soft, high pitch, moderate duration): heard over liver, heart, spleen, or muscles
    d) Flatness (extreme dullness, soft, high-pitched, short duration): heard over muscle

e) Tympany (drumlike, loud, high pitch, moderate duration): heard over air-filled stomach

4. Abnormal findings
   a) Hyperresonance over an adult lung may indicate emphysema or pneumothorax.
   b) Dullness over adult lung may be a sign of pneumonia, hemothorax (blood in pleural cavity), or tumor.
   c) Flatness not over muscle may indicate pleural effusion (fluid in pleural cavity).

5. Assessment of diaphragmatic excursion
   a) Purpose: to assess diaphragmatic movement
   b) Procedure: normally performed on posterior thorax
      (1) Instruct client to take a deep breath and hold it.
      (2) Percuss down the posterior thorax along the scapular line until dullness is found, indicating the border of the diaphragm.
      (3) Mark on each side of spine point at which dullness begins (diaphragm usually slightly higher on right).
      (4) Instruct client to exhale and wait before inhaling.
      (5) Percuss above previously marked point of dullness to detect new point of dullness.
      (6) Mark new point of dullness.
      (7) Measure and record distance (usually 3–6 cm) between first and second marks.

E. Auscultation of the lungs
   1. Purposes: to assess breath sounds and lung condition and to detect airflow obstructions
   2. Special equipment: stethoscope with appropriate size chestpiece
   3. Stethoscope placement and sequence
      a) Warm stethoscope with hands.
      b) Place diaphragm of stethoscope firmly on skin.
         (1) Do not place over clothing.
         (2) If auscultating over hair, wet hair first (hair can alter breath sounds).
      c) Instruct the client to breathe a little more deeply than normal, but not too quickly, with the mouth open.
      d) Be alert for signs of hyperventilation and stop if client feels faint or lightheaded.
      e) Auscultate apices and posterior, lateral, and anterior chest.
         (1) Follow the same sequence used for percussion (see section III,D,2 of this chapter).
         (2) Listen to 1 full breath in each location.
         (3) Compare corresponding areas.

4. Breath sounds
    a) Normal breath sounds
        (1) Vesicular breath sounds: caused by the movement of air into alveoli
            (a) Low pitch, soft intensity (like a "breeze")
            (b) Heard over most of the lung
            (c) Best heard during inspiration
            (d) Longer duration (2.5–3 times as long) during inspiration than expiration
        (2) Bronchovesicular breath sounds: occur when air moves through the smaller bronchi and bronchioles
            (a) Equal duration during inspiration and expiration, medium pitch, medium intensity
            (b) Heard in areas of bronchi at first and second intercostal spaces anteriorly and between the scapulae posteriorly
            (c) Between vesicular breath sounds and bronchial sounds in duration, intensity, and pitch
        (3) Bronchial (tracheal) breath sounds: caused by air moving through the bronchi
            (a) High-pitched, loud intensity
            (b) Heard over the trachea
            (c) Longer during expiration
            (d) Pause between inspiration and expiration
    b) Abnormal (adventitious) or altered breath sounds
        (1) Bronchial or bronchovesicular sounds: caused by fluid in the lungs
            (a) Heard over peripheral lung
            (b) May indicate pneumonia or pleurisy
        (2) Absent or decreased breath sounds: may be a sign of obstruction, pneumothorax, or emphysema
        (3) Crackles (rales or crepitations)
            (a) Classified as fine (resembles the sound produced when rubbing hairs together near the ear) to coarse (a gurgling sound)
            (b) Caused by air passing through secretions or diminished airways
            (c) May indicate asthma, bronchitis, congestive heart failure (CHF), or an interstitial lung disorder
            (d) Pathologic crackles: will not clear with coughing
        (4) Wheezes
            (a) Continuous, high-pitched whistling sound
            (b) Caused by air passing through narrowed airways
            (c) May indicate asthma, bronchitis, croup, CHF, or tumor
            (d) Usually occur during expiration but may be apparent during inspiration as well
            (e) May clear with coughing

(5) Rhonchi
    (a) Sonorous quality: continuous, low-pitched rattling in the throat resembling snoring
    (b) Caused by air moving through fluid-filled airways
    (c) May indicate infection
    (d) Usually heard during expiration but may occur during inspiration
    (e) Usually clear with coughing

(6) Pleural friction rubs
    (a) Creaking, grating sound
    (b) Caused by the rubbing together of inflamed pleural surfaces
    (c) May indicate pneumonia, tuberculosis, or pulmonary embolism
    (d) Usually heard during inspiration and expiration but may be heard only during inspiration or with increased intensity during inspiration
    (e) Best heard in lower anterolateral thorax

(7) Stridor
    (a) High-pitched, crowing sound
    (b) Caused by partial obstruction of upper airway
    (c) May indicate croup (in children), aspiration of foreign object, or tumor
    (d) Heard during inspiration

5. Vocal resonance
  a) Sounds heard through the stethoscope when the client speaks
  b) Testing for vocal resonance: when abnormality has been detected through inspection, palpation, percussion, or auscultation
    (1) Ask client to say the words "one, two, three" or "ninety-nine."
      (a) Normal: muffled, indistinct sound
      (b) Abnormal: words heard clearly (bronchophony)
    (2) Ask client to say "eeee."
      (a) Normal: muffled "eeee" sound
      (b) Abnormal: "ay" sound heard; voice nasal (egophony)
    (3) Ask client to whisper "one, two, three" or "ninety-nine."
      (a) Normal: barely audible sound
      (b) Abnormal: whispered words heard distinctly (whispered pectoriloquy)
  c) Abnormal findings indicate consolidation of lung tissue.

6. Modifications for pregnant clients, infants, children and adolescents, and the elderly (see sections I,B; II,B; III,B; and IV,B of Chapter 3)

F. Diagnostic tests
   1. Chest x-ray
   2. Arterial blood gas analysis
   3. Red blood cell count
   4. Hemoglobin
   5. Sputum culture and sensitivity
   6. Pulmonary function tests
   7. Tuberculosis skin test

IV. Essential nursing care for client with suspected asthma

See text pages
_____

A. Nursing assessment
   1. Gather relevant health history information (same as section I of this chapter).
   2. Perform physical assessment (same as section III of this chapter).
   3. Assist with diagnostic tests.

B. Nursing diagnoses
   1. Ineffective airway clearance related to exposure to respiratory irritants as revealed by auscultation of the thorax
   2. High risk for altered respiratory status related to knowledge deficit concerning asthma triggers
   3. High risk for noncompliance related to knowledge deficit concerning disease treatment
   4. Anxiety related to fear of asthma attacks as expressed by client

C. Nursing implementation (intervention)
   1. Explain lung function and the effects of asthma on breathing to the client.
   2. Teach client about asthma triggers and how to avoid them.
   3. Teach client to recognize the early warning signs of asthma.
   4. Stress the importance of taking daily medication and working with physician, family, and health care workers to control asthma.
   5. Instruct the client to report any changes in his/her condition to physician.
   6. Refer client to an asthma education program and support group.

D. Nursing evaluation
   1. Client demonstrates through verbalization an awareness of asthma triggers and avoids them.
   2. Client demonstrates through verbalization an understanding of the signs and symptoms of an asthma attack.

I. Relevant health history	II. Anatomy and physiology	III. Assessment techniques	IV. Essential nursing care for client with suspected asthma

3. Client takes medication as prescribed.
4. Client monitors his/her condition and reports any changes to the physician.
5. Client demonstrates increased confidence about his/her ability to control the disease.

1. What important client-centered role can the nurse play in preventing lung disease from environmental respiratory irritants such as cigarette smoke, radon, and pollens?

   a. Client advocate
   b. Client educator
   c. Hospice nurse
   d. Critical care nurse

2. After auscultating the chest of an 18-year-old male, the nurse writes: "Pleural friction rub heard at the right fifth intercostal space at the MCL." This statement means the rub is heard on the right side of the chest:

   a. Between the fifth and sixth ribs on the line that runs vertically through the middle of the sternum.
   b. Between the fourth and fifth ribs on the line that runs vertically through the middle of the clavicle.
   c. Between the fifth and sixth ribs on the line that runs vertically through the middle of the clavicle.
   d. Between the fifth and sixth ribs on the line that runs horizontally through the middle of the clavicle.

3. The nurse is performing a chest assessment of a 38-year-old male client. The nurse observes that the chest expands equally and symmetrically, and the ratio of the anteroposterior diameter to the transverse diameter is 1:2. These are characteristics of a:

   a. Normal chest.
   b. Barrel chest.
   c. Flail chest.
   d. Funnel chest.

4. A female client is 30 years old, has mild scoliosis, and is 7 months pregnant. She states she is short of breath after climbing a flight of stairs. The most likely reason for this client's dyspnea after climbing stairs is:

   a. The uterus with the growing fetus forces the diaphragm downward.
   b. Her oxygenation and ventilation needs are increased due to the pregnancy.
   c. Her scoliosis decreases alveolar gas exchange of both lungs.
   d. Total lung capacity decreases after 30 years of age.

5. The nurse is checking vital signs at 4 A.M. One of her clients, a 75-year-old female with diabetes, is breathing very deeply at 44 breaths per minute. This type of respiratory pattern is:

   a. Paroxysmal nocturnal dyspnea.
   b. Biot's breathing.
   c. Kussmaul's respirations.
   d. Cheyne-Stokes respirations.

6. A 60-year-old retired coal miner has been diagnosed with chronic obstructive pulmonary disease (COPD). He states that he becomes short of breath after climbing 3 steps. He must sleep upright in his recliner. Physical assessment findings include: respirations 24 per minute, shallow; pursed-lip breathing; use of intercostal and neck muscles on every respiration. His laboratory values for arterial blood gases are: PO_2=69mm Hg; PCO_2=50mm Hg. An accurate nursing diagnosis for this client is:

   a. Activity intolerance related to dyspnea on climbing stairs.
   b. COPD related to exposure to coal dust.
   c. Ineffective airway clearance related to COPD shown by use of accessory muscles for breathing.
   d. Ineffective breathing pattern related to increased PO_2 and decreased PCO_2.

7. Of the following choices, the *priority* nursing diagnosis for the client described in the preceding question is:

   a. Activity intolerance related to dyspnea on climbing stairs.
   b. High risk for impaired physical mobility related to chronic illness.

The Respiratory System   113

c. Impaired gas exchange related to decreased arterial blood oxygen concentration.

d. Altered nutrition, more than body requirements, related to inactivity.

8. The nurse palpates the chest to collect assessment data on the:

a. Presence or absence of fremitus.
b. Location of vesicular breath sounds.
c. Quality of crackles or wheezes.
d. Degree of intercostal retraction.

9. The nurse is percussing the posterior intercostal spaces of the chest of a 4-year-old boy. She is listening for the normal percussion tone of:

a. Resonance.
b. Tympany.
c. Dullness.
d. Hyperresonance.

10. Using the stethoscope, the nurse listens to the lungs of a 23-year-old man. While auscultating at the right and left second intercostal space between the scapulae, the nurse hears breath sounds with equal phases of inspiration and expiration and of medium pitch and intensity. She knows these breath sounds are:

a. Normal bronchovesicular sounds.
b. Abnormal bronchovesicular sounds.
c. Normal bronchial sounds.
d. Abnormal bronchial sounds.

11. As the nurse auscultates the lungs of a 27-year-old client with asthma, the nurse hears a continuous, high-pitched whistling sound during expiration in all lobes of both lungs. The nurse has heard:

a. Rhonchi.
b. Crackles.
c. Wheezes.
d. Pleural friction rubs.

12. Crackles in the lower lobes and a copious amount of frothy, blood-streaked, or reddish brown sputum may indicate:

a. A normal finding.
b. A sinus infection with a postnasal drip.
c. An upper respiratory infection.
d. Pulmonary edema or pneumonia.

ANSWERS

1. **Correct answer is b.** Educating clients to avoid exposure to respiratory irritants by nonuse, removal, exclusion, or wearing protective masks and clothing is a crucial client-centered role that will lessen clients' risks of contracting lung disease.

   a. The nurse may function as a client advocate by informing companies and testifying in court on the health hazards of their products to groups of clients, but client education is crucial to primary prevention of lung disease.
   c. Hospice nurses care for the terminally ill.
   d. Critical care nurses care for clients who are seriously ill in the hospital. Their focus is prevention of further complications from an illness.

2. **Correct answer is c.** The fifth intercostal space is between the fifth and sixth ribs. The MCL is the midclavicular line. It lies perpendicular to the middle of the clavicle and runs vertically down the rib cage.

   a. The midsternal line runs vertically through the middle of the sternum.
   b. The fourth intercostal space is between the fourth and fifth ribs.
   d. The MCL runs vertically through the middle of the clavicle.

3. **Correct answer is a.** Symmetrical chest expansion and a 1:2 anteroposterior to transverse diameter are 2 characteristics of a normal chest.

   b. A barrel chest is characterized by an increased anteroposterior diameter. The ratio of the anteroposterior diameter to the transverse diameter approaches 1:1. This is common in chronic obstructive pulmonary disease (COPD).

c. A flail chest describes paradoxical chest movement on inspiration and expiration due to a segment of unattached, fractured ribs.

d. A funnel chest, or pectus excavatum, describes a depression at the lower sternum. Depending on the depth of the depression, this may interfere with respiration.

4. **Correct answer is b.** The growing fetus increases the client's oxygenation and ventilation needs. Also, the pregnant uterus in the third trimester pushes upward on the diaphragm and crowds the lungs and other internal organs.

a. The diaphragm is forced upward, not downward.

c. Mild scoliosis may slightly decrease tidal volume, but does not impair gas exchange at the alveolar level to the point of causing dyspnea on exertion.

d. Total lung capacity does not necessarily decrease after 30 years of age. With sufficient aerobic exercise, total lung capacity can increase after 30 years of age.

5. **Correct answer is c.** Kussmaul's respirations are very deep with a rapid respiratory rate and are seen during episodes of diabetic acidosis and in severe renal disease.

a. Paroxysmal nocturnal dyspnea is sudden, periodic episodes of shortness of breath occurring at night, usually a short time after lying down.

b. Irregular respirations with periods of apnea characterize Biot's breathing, which occurs with brain damage and respiratory depression.

d. Cheyne-Stokes respirations occur in central nervous (CNS) system disorders and extreme intoxication. Their pattern is cyclic with slow, shallow respirations increasing to faster, deeper respirations, then decreasing again in rate and depth until a period of apnea occurs. The pattern then repeats in the same manner.

6. **Correct answer is a.** This client cannot tolerate the activity of climbing stairs without becoming dyspneic.

b. COPD is an accurate *medical* diagnosis.

c. No data support ineffective airway clearance. In addition, the use of accessory muscles for breathing is not a defining characteristic of ineffective airway clearance.

d. Pursed-lip breathing is an ineffective breathing pattern, but his PO_2 is decreased and PCO_2 is increased.

7. **Correct answer is c.** Impaired gas exchange exists at the alveolar level, and his PO_2 is decreased. This is the priority nursing diagnosis because severely impaired gas exchange is incompatible with life.

a. This is an accurate nursing diagnosis based on the data given, but it is not life-threatening.

b. A high risk nursing diagnosis is one that has not actually occurred, but is likely to occur with a given set of circumstances. The client already has impaired physical mobility.

d. No data are given on his nutritional intake nor the degree of his daily activity/inactivity.

8. **Correct answer is a.** Fremitus, a normal finding, is a vibration caused by the client's voice and felt by the palmar surface of the nurse's hands on palpation of the chest.

b. Auscultation of the chest is used to locate vesicular breath sounds.

c. The quality of crackles or wheezes are determined by auscultation of the chest.

d. The nurse inspects the chest for the degree of intercostal retraction.

9. **Correct answer is d.** Hyperresonance, a booming sound, is the normal percussion tone of a child's lungs. Hyperresonance is abnormal in the adult's lungs and may be heard in clients with COPD.

   a. Resonance, a hollow sound, is the normal percussion tone in the lungs of an adult.
   b. Tympany, a drumlike sound, is the normal percussion tone heard over the gastric air bubble of the stomach.
   c. Dullness, a thudlike sound, is the normal percussion tone heard over a solid tissue, such as the liver, spleen, or heart.

10. **Correct answer is a.** The nurse is listening to an area where bronchovesicular sounds, breath sounds with equal inspiratory and expiratory phases, are normal.

   b. In pathologic conditions, bronchovesicular sounds may occur outside of their designated chest locations, thus becoming abnormal sounds. These sounds, however, were heard in the expected location.
   c. Normal bronchial sounds occur over the mainstem bronchi and the trachea.
   d. Abnormal bronchial sounds may be heard outside of their designated chest area in pathologic conditions, such as pneumonia. They are high-pitched and loud, however, and are longer during expiration.

11. **Correct answer is c.** Wheezes, high pitched whistling or musical sounds, are caused by air flowing through the narrowed airways of constricted bronchioles.

   a. Rhonchi are low-pitched, sonorous sounds caused by air moving through fluid-filled airways.
   b. Crackles are medium-pitched sounds caused by air moving through secretions and/or diminished airways. They range in quality from fine (popping) to coarse (gurgling).
   d. Pleural friction rubs, which disappear when the client holds his/her breath, are grating sounds caused by inflamed pleura rubbing together.

12. **Correct answer is d.** Fluid in the alveoli and bronchioles will cause crackles and, sometimes, blood-tinged sputum. Pulmonary edema and pneumonia have different etiologies, but both are characterized by excess fluid in the lungs.

   a. Clear to white sputum and vesicular breath sounds with no crackles are normal findings.
   b. A sinus infection with a postnasal drip may cause coughing but no abnormal lung sounds such as crackles on auscultation.
   c. An upper respiratory infection is characterized by copious nasal discharge, swollen nasal turbinates, watery eyes, and at times, a sore throat.

7

The Cardiovascular System

OVERVIEW

I. Relevant health history
  A. Current status
  B. Past status
  C. Family history
  D. Risk factors: cardiac disease

II. Anatomy and physiology
  A. The heart
  B. The great vessels and blood circulation
  C. The cardiac cycle
  D. The cardiac conduction system

III. Assessment techniques
  A. Approach
  B. General inspection
  C. Inspection and palpation of the precordium
  D. Percussion of the precordium
  E. Auscultation of the precordium
  F. Assessment of jugular venous pressure and pulse
  G. Assessment of peripheral arterial pulses

IV. Essential nursing care for client with chest pain
  A. Nursing assessment
  B. Nursing diagnoses
  C. Nursing implementation (intervention)
  D. Nursing evaluation

NURSING HIGHLIGHTS

1. Basic auscultation skills (recognizing normal heart sounds and splitting) require much experience and practice. Recognizing abnormal signs (murmurs, clicks, snaps, friction rubs, gallops) requires even greater skill. The nurse should not expect to attain the higher level until thoroughly experienced with basic auscultation.

2. The most important signs and symptoms of cardiac disease to note during history and physical examination are chest pain, dyspnea with or without coughing, dizziness, edema, palpitations, fatigue, and cyanosis evident in skin, nail beds, and mucous membranes.

3. Commonly used drugs that can cause cardiovascular adverse effects include tricyclic antidepressants, the antineoplastics daunorubicin and doxorubicin hydrochloride, diazepam, conjugated estrogens, vasopressin, indomethacin, theophylline, bethanechol chloride, hydralazine hydrochloride, and phenytoin sodium.

GLOSSARY

aneurysm—localized dilatation or weakening of the wall of a blood vessel

angina pectoris—chest pain that may radiate to left arm, neck, or jaw usually caused by inadequate oxygen supply to the myocardium

heave—upward rising of chest that can be palpated, caused by cardiac disorder; also called a lift

myocardial infarction (MI)—occlusion of a coronary artery resulting in the death of heart tissue

regurgitation—backward flow of blood through a defective heart valve

septal defect—abnormal, usually congenital, opening in the wall separating the chambers of the heart

stenosis—the narrowing of an opening or passageway in a body structure

thrill—a palpable murmur; feels like the fine vibration felt on the throat of purring cat

ENHANCED OUTLINE

See text pages
_____

I. Relevant health history

A. Current status
1. Does the client have chest pain or discomfort in the chest (see Nurse Alert, "Assessing Chest Pain")?
   a) Description (e.g., type, location, radiation of pain)
   b) Duration (e.g., length of time client has had pain, length of individual attack)
   c) Associated symptoms (e.g., dizziness, palpitations, pallor, cyanosis)
   d) Palliative or provocative factors (e.g., strenuous activity, rest)
2. Does the client have shortness of breath? Is it accompanied by a cough?
   a) Timing of attack
   b) Associated symptoms (e.g., cough, syncope)
3. Does the client ever feel dizzy when changing positions?

4. Does the client have signs of edema?
    a) Description (e.g., feet or ankles swell, shoes or rings feel tight)
    b) Duration (length of time client has had edema)
5. Does the client's heart seem to pound, race, flutter, or skip beats?
6. Does the client experience frequent fatigue?
    a) Description of fatigue-producing activities (including length of time client can perform activity before getting tired)
    b) Behaviors that relieve the fatigue (e.g., stopping, resting)
    c) Associated symptoms (e.g., pain, shortness of breath)
7. What prescription or over-the-counter (OTC) medications does the client take?
8. Does the client use salt, tobacco, alcohol, or caffeine products?
    a) Amount and frequency
    b) Effects with use (e.g., edema, tachycardia)

B. Past status
1. Was the client born with a heart defect? If so, when and how was it treated?
2. Has the client ever had rheumatic fever or rheumatic heart disease?
    a) Time of occurrence
    b) Residual problems
3. Has the client ever been told he/she has a heart murmur?
4. Has the client been diagnosed with hypertension, hyperlipidemia, or diabetes mellitus?
    a) Time of diagnosis
    b) Treatments
5. Has the client ever experienced any of the following symptoms?
    a) Chest pain
    b) Shortness of breath
    c) Diaphoresis (sweating) without exertion
    d) Fainting or dizziness
    e) Foot or ankle swelling
    f) Unusual fatigue
    g) Periods of confusion
    h) Palpitations
    i) Bluish discoloration of skin
6. Has the client had any invasive procedure, including dental work, within the last month?

C. Family history: Has anyone in the client's family been diagnosed with cardiovascular disease, diabetes mellitus, or hyperlipidemia?

D. Risk factors: cardiac disease
1. Heredity: cardiac disease or hyperlipidemia occurring in blood relative before age 55
2. Race: higher incidence among blacks
3. Sex: More males than females develop cardiac disease; after menopause, women's risk increases dramatically.
4. Age: increased risk with age

5. Hypertension: blood pressure consistently exceeding 140/90 mm Hg
6. Cigarette smoking
7. Hyperlipidemia (total cholesterol above 180 mg/dl)
8. Diabetes mellitus
9. Oral contraceptive use
10. Left ventricular hypertrophy (LVH)
11. Contributing factors include obesity, inactivity, stressful lifestyle, diet high in cholesterol and saturated fats

II. Anatomy and physiology

See text pages

_____

A. The heart: muscular organ with 4 chambers
   1. Position
      a) Heart is located in thoracic cavity within mediastinum, between second and sixth ribs; usually lies obliquely with one-third to the right of midsternal line and two-thirds to the left of it.
      b) Position varies with build of individual.
   2. Basic structure
      a) Base: superior portion of heart, lying behind superior portion of sternal body at about T2; includes atria
      b) Apex: inferior portion of heart pointing down and left, normally lies at the midclavicular line in the fifth left intercostal space
      c) Heart wall (3 layers): endocardium (inner layer), myocardium (muscular middle layer), epicardium (outermost layer, continuous with pericardial lining)
      d) Pericardium: fibrous sac encasing heart
         (1) 2 layers: outer layer continuous with covering of great vessels; inner layer continuous with epicardium
         (2) Serous fluid between layers
   3. Heart chambers: work together with valves to send blood through heart
      a) Ventricles (left and right)
         (1) These thick-walled chambers are inferior to corresponding atria.
         (2) Left and right ventricles are separated by interventricular septum.
         (3) They contract during systole and relax during diastole.
         (4) Left ventricular wall is thicker than right.
      b) Atria (left and right)
         (1) These thin-walled chambers are superior to corresponding ventricles.
         (2) Left and right atria are separated by interatrial septum.
         (3) Atria act as reservoirs for blood from veins between contractions.

4. Heart valves: permit one-way flow of blood through heart
  a) Atrioventricular (AV) valves: between atria and ventricles
    (1) Tricuspid valve: right AV valve
    (2) Mitral (bicuspid) valve: left AV valve
  b) Semilunar (SL) valves: between ventricles and great vessels, aorta and pulmonary artery
    (1) Pulmonic valve: right SL valve, between right ventricle and pulmonary artery
    (2) Aortic valve: left SL valve, between left ventricle and aorta

B. The great vessels and blood circulation
  1. Great vessels
    a) Superior and inferior vena cavae, pulmonary artery, pulmonary veins, aorta
    b) Enter heart at base (top)
  2. Circulation process
    a) From body, superior vena cava (upper body) and inferior vena cava (lower body) return deoxygenated blood to right atrium.
    b) Deoxygenated blood enters right ventricle.
    c) Deoxygenated blood enters pulmonary artery; artery bifurcates to right and left leading to lungs (where blood is oxygenated).
    d) From lungs, pulmonary veins return oxygenated blood to left atrium.
    e) Oxygenated blood enters left ventricle.
    f) Blood enters aorta, which curves upward over heart, then backward and down, returning oxygenated blood to body.
      (1) 3 aortic branches supply brain, upper extremities, and upper chest.

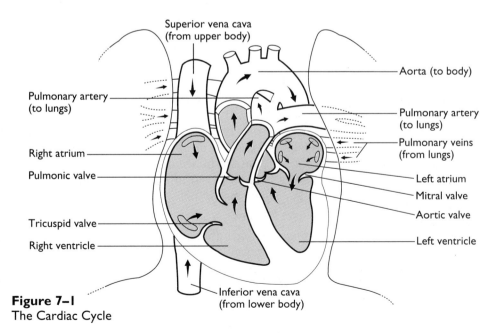

Figure 7–1
The Cardiac Cycle

(2) Aorta travels down through thorax and abdomen to supply organs and tissues of lower chest and abdomen.

(3) Aorta divides into iliac arteries, which divide into femoral arteries, to supply lower extremities.

3. Types of blood vessels

    a) Arteries have thick, muscular walls; carry blood away from heart.

    b) Arterioles receive blood from arteries; have thinner walls that can constrict and dilate.

    c) Capillaries receive blood from arterioles; through their very thin walls blood and tissues exchange nutrients and gases.

    d) Venules gather blood from capillaries.

    e) Veins return blood from venules to heart.

C. The cardiac cycle: systole and diastole

1. Systole: ventricular contraction that forces blood out of the heart

    a) Blood ejected from the ventricles, AV valves close, producing first heart sound (S_1).

    b) With rising pressure SL valves open and blood is ejected into aorta.

    c) Ventricle relaxes, pressure drops, and SL valves close, producing second heart sound (S_2) at beginning of diastole.

2. Diastole: ventricular relaxation that allows heart to fill with blood

    a) AV valves open, allowing blood to flow from atria into ventricles (S_3 may be heard in children, young adults, and in the last trimester of pregnancy).

    b) Atria contract to eject remaining blood (S_4 sometimes heard immediately before S_1).

3. Splitting of heart sounds: caused by delay of events on right side of heart

    a) Events on right side of heart occur slightly later than comparable events on left side because right side pressure is lower.

    b) S_1 has 2 components, but usually heard as 1 sound: M_1, mitral valve closure (louder), and T_1, tricuspid valve closure; S_1 splitting best heard at lower left sternal border but may be undetectable.

    c) S_2 has 2 components, but usually heard as 1 sound: A_2, aortic valve closure (louder) and then P_2, pulmonic valve closure; S_2 splitting best heard on inspiration and more easily heard than S_1 splitting.

D. The cardiac conduction system: electric impulses that regulate cardiac cycle

1. Sinoatrial (SA) node: pacemaker of heart

    a) Node located in right atrium near opening of superior vena cava.

    b) It fires to stimulate atrial contraction about 60–100 times a minute.

    c) Impulse travels to atrioventricular node.

2. Atrioventricular (AV) node
   a) Node located in right atrium just above tricuspid valve.
   b) Impulse delayed briefly here, then passes through His's bundle and Purkinje's fibers, stimulating ventricular contraction.
3. Electrocardiogram (ECG or EKG): records electrical impulses
   a) P wave—spread of SA impulse through atria
   b) QRS complex—spread of AV impulse through ventricles
   c) T wave—ventricular recovery

III. Assessment techniques

See text pages

_____

A. Approach
   1. Provide privacy.
   2. Keep room at a comfortable temperature.
   3. Select quiet environment for auscultation of heart sounds.
   4. Use proper client position: supine, head of bed elevated about 30° (up to 45° for clients with breathing problems).

B. General inspection
   1. Note general appearance: Note any deviations from norm.
   2. Assess vital signs (see section I,F of Chapter 2).
   3. Note any abnormalities in shape of thorax (see section III,B,1,c of Chapter 6).
   4. Note any pallor or cyanosis of skin; clubbing of fingers (see section III,D of Chapter 4).
   5. Note appearance and location of any lesions, especially on lower extremities.

C. Inspection and palpation of the precordium: to assess normal and abnormal pulsations
   1. Technique
      a) Client should be supine with nurse at right side (if right-handed); with obese or large-breasted client, inspection may be easier with client sitting.
      b) Tangential lighting aids inspection process.
      c) Use finger pads for palpation.
      d) Assess 5 areas of precordium in systematic manner.
      e) Pulsations in some precordial areas are normal in children and thin adults.
   2. Aortic area: second right intercostal space at sternal border
      a) Normal findings: no pulsation
      b) Abnormal findings: Pulsations may indicate aortic aneurysm or aortic regurgitation; palpable S_2 may indicate systemic hypertension; thrill may indicate aortic stenosis.
   3. Pulmonic area: second left intercostal space at sternal border
      a) Normal findings: no pulsation
      b) Abnormal findings: Pulsations or thrills may indicate pulmonary hypertension, mitral stenosis, atrial septal defect, pulmonic valve stenosis; palpable S_2 may indicate pulmonary hypertension.

4. Left sternal border (right ventricular): third, fourth, and fifth left intercostal spaces
    a) Normal findings: no pulsation
    b) Abnormal findings: Pulsations or heaves may indicate right ventricular hypertrophy caused by pulmonary hypertension or pulmonary valve disease; thrill may indicate ventricular septal defect or pulmonary valve disease.
5. Apical area (left ventricular): at midclavicular line at about fifth left intercostal space
    a) Normal findings: visible pulsation of apical impulse
        (1) Assess location.
        (2) Assess diameter: should be ≤2.5 cm.
        (3) Assess amplitude: should be like a light tap.
        (4) Assess duration: should be sustained during first two-thirds or less of systole.

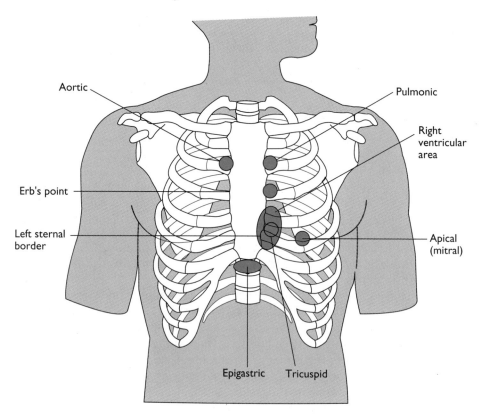

Figure 7–2
Inspection, Palpation, and Auscultation of the Precordium

b) Abnormal findings: Abnormally forceful or lengthy pulsation, displaced pulsation, or one with increased diameter may indicate left ventricular hypertrophy (LVH) or ventricular aneurysm.

6. Epigastric area: base of sternum
   a) Normal findings: No pulsation, although pulsation may be normal after exercise in some individuals.
   b) Abnormal findings: Bounding pulsations may indicate aortic aneurysm, aortic regurgitation, fever, anemia, thyrotoxicosis.

D. Percussion of the precordium
   1. Estimate of cardiac size can be made through percussion; procedures such as chest x-ray are more accurate.
   2. With client supine, begin at anterior left axillary line and percuss toward sternum in fifth intercostal space; dullness should locate left border of heart at midclavicular line in fifth intercostal space.

E. Auscultation of the precordium
   1. Sites: may be named for underlying structure or position
      a) Aortic (second right intercostal space)
      b) Pulmonic (second left intercostal space)
      c) Erb's point (third left intercostal space)
      d) Tricuspid (fourth left intercostal space)
      e) Mitral (apical)
   2. Positioning: Auscultate all 5 areas with diaphragm and bell of stethoscope with client in 3 positions.
      a) Client supine with nurse to the right (if right-handed)
      b) Seated and leaning forward, breath held after expiration
      c) Left lateral recumbent
   3. Techniques
      a) Hold warmed chestpiece of stethoscope against skin (wet chest hair if necessary).
         (1) Press diaphragm firmly on skin; best for high-pitched sounds (e.g., S_1, S_2, aortic regurgitation).
         (2) Rest bell lightly on skin; best for low-pitched sounds (e.g., S_3, S_4, murmurs).
      b) Auscultate in unhurried manner and listen selectively for each component.
         (1) Listen to all 5 auscultation sites, in sequence (beginning at apex and working to base).
         (2) Listen for several cycles.
         (3) Listen for rate, rhythm, pitch, and intensity of sound.
         (4) Listen for S_1: intensity, splitting, effects of respiration (have client exhale and hold breath and then inhale and hold breath).
         (5) Listen for S_2: intensity, splitting, effects of respiration (see section III,E,3,b,4 of this chapter).
         (6) Concentrate on systole: Check for extra sounds or murmurs.
         (7) Concentrate on diastole: Check for extra sounds or murmurs.

4. Normal findings
   a) S_1 normally louder than S_2 at the apex and lower sternal border; S_2 louder at the base.
   b) Split S_1 may be heard along lower left sternal border.
   c) Split S_2 is normal at the left second and third intercostal space on inspiration, but should disappear on expiration (in children and young adults split S_2 may continue on expiration).
   d) Palpating the carotid artery simultaneously with auscultation can help identify S_1, which is almost simultaneous with the upstroke of the pulse beat.
   e) Diastolic pause between S_2 and S_1 normally longer than the systolic pause between S_1 and S_2; there should be no other sounds during these pauses.
5. Abnormal findings
   a) S_1 abnormalities
      (1) Accentuated, diminished, or inaudible S_1
      (2) S_1 of varying intensity
      (3) Split S_1 heard at apex
   b) S_2 abnormalities
      (1) Accentuated, diminished, or inaudible S_2
      (2) Wide splitting: increased split, especially on inspiration
      (3) Fixed splitting: increased split that does not vary with respiration
      (4) Reversed/paradoxical splitting: splitting that appears on expiration and disappears on inspiration
      (5) $P_2 \geq A_2$
      (6) Decreased or absent P_2
   c) Extra systolic sounds: Note location, timing, intensity, pitch.
      (1) Early systolic ejection sounds: high pitch, sharp quality
      (2) Systolic clicks: usually midsystolic to late systolic, high-pitched, caused by mitral valve dysfunction
   d) Extra diastolic sounds: Note location, timing, intensity, pitch, effect of respiration on sound.
      (1) Opening snap: heard early in diastole (just after S_2) medial to apex, involves mitral or tricuspid valve dysfunction
      (2) S_3 (ventricular gallop): low-pitched, early to mid-diastole; may be heard normally in children, young adults, and women in third trimester of pregnancy; otherwise abnormal
      (3) S_4 (atrial gallop): low-pitched, low-intensity sound; heard best at apex; immediately precedes S_1; may be considered normal in some adults over 40, especially after exercise; otherwise abnormal

(4) Summation gallop: both S$_3$ and S$_4$ heard along with S$_1$ and S$_2$; quadruple rhythm
- e) Other extra heart sounds
    - (1) Pericardial friction rub: high-pitched scratchy or scraping sound at left sternal border caused by inflammation of pericardium
    - (2) Venous hum: low-pitched continuous humming or roaring heard in internal jugular vein
- f) Murmurs
    - (1) Blowing or rasping sound caused by turbulence of blood flow because of regurgitation or stenosis
    - (2) Identification
        - (a) Location
            - (i) Area of greatest intensity
            - (ii) Areas of radiation
        - (b) Timing
            - (i) Systolic (between S$_1$ and S$_2$), diastolic (between S$_2$ and S$_1$), or continuous (heard in both)
            - (ii) Can divide further into midsystolic, pansystolic (through entire period, also called holosystolic), late systolic; early diastolic, mid-diastolic, late diastolic (presystolic)
        - (c) Quality
            - (i) Blowing
            - (ii) Harsh
            - (iii) Rumbling
            - (iv) Musical
        - (d) Pitch
            - (i) High: heard only with diaphragm
            - (ii) Low: heard only with bell
            - (iii) Medium: heard with both diaphragm and bell
        - (e) Pattern or shape: intensity over time
            - (i) Crescendo: grows louder
            - (ii) Decrescendo: grows softer
            - (iii) Crescendo-decrescendo: rises in intensity, then falls
            - (iv) Plateau: same intensity throughout
        - (f) Intensity: Use 6-point grading system.
            - (i) Grade I: very faint, barely audible
            - (ii) Grade II: quiet, but easily audible with stethoscope held on chest
            - (iii) Grade III: moderately loud
            - (iv) Grade IV: loud, associated with thrill
            - (v) Grade V: very loud, audible with stethoscope partly off chest, thrill easily palpable
            - (vi) Grade VI: extremely loud, audible with stethoscope held over but not touching chest, palpable thrill

F. Assessment of jugular venous pressure and pulse
   1. Measure jugular venous pressure.
      a) Position client supine with the trunk elevated 30°–45°; the client's head should be turned slightly away from the examiner.
      b) Use tangential lighting.
      c) Assess jugular (central) venous pressure.
         (1) Locate angle of Louis (sternal angle).
         (2) Note highest level of visible pulsation in internal jugular vein.
         (3) Measure vertical distance from this point to angle of Louis; normal distance is ≤2 cm.
   2. Assess jugular venous pulse in right internal jugular vein.
      a) Consists of 3 ascending and 2 descending components.
         (1) The a wave: occurs just before S_1 and is produced by right atrial contraction; identify by palpating carotid artery (wave occurs just before carotid pulsation) or listening to heart sounds
         (2) The c wave: occurs at end of S_1 and is the result of carotid artery pulsation; small and rarely seen
         (3) The x descent: follows c wave and is produced by atrial relaxation
         (4) The v wave: indicates filling in of vena cava and right atrium as tricuspid valve closes
         (5) The y descent: follows v wave, occurring early in diastole just after S_2 when tricuspid valve opens
      b) Assess for abnormalities: absent or unusually prominent waves.

G. Assessment of peripheral arterial pulses: Palpate all pulses and auscultate carotid and apical pulses as well.
   1. Techniques
      a) Use pads of index and middle fingers.
      b) Press gently; excessive pressure may obliterate pulsation.
      c) Identify pulse rate, rhythm, quality at each site (see section I,F of Chapter 2 for pulse assessment information).
      d) Work from head to toe, comparing pulses side to side.
   2. Arterial pulse points
      a) Temporal pulse: Position fingers lateral to eye orbit, anterior to tragus of ear.
      b) Carotid pulse
         (1) Position fingers just medial to trachea and below angle of jaw.
         (2) Palpate only 1 carotid artery at a time.
         (3) Place bell of stethoscope on skin over carotid artery as client holds breath to listen for bruits.

c) Brachial pulse: Position fingers medial to biceps tendon on anterior surface of elbow joint.

d) Radial pulse: Position fingers just below thumb on palmar surface of the wrist, with the wrist relaxed and slightly flexed.

e) Femoral pulse: Position fingers firmly in the groin area just below the midpoint of the inguinal ligament.

f) Popliteal pulse: Position fingers firmly in popliteal fossa of the back of the flexed knee.

g) Dorsalis pedis pulse: Position fingers on medial dorsum of foot with toes pointed down; pulse may be absent in elderly clients or congenitally absent.

h) Posterior tibial pulse: Position fingers behind and slightly below malleolus of ankle with toes pointed down; may be congenitally absent.

3. Normal findings
   a) Pulse rate should be 60–100 beats/minute in adults.
   b) Rhythm should be regular.
   c) Pulse should be easily palpated and obliterated only with strong pressure.

4. Abnormal findings (see section I,F,2,e of Chapter 2)
   a) Abnormalities of rate: tachycardia, bradycardia
   b) Abnormalities of rhythm: dysrhythmia, bigeminal pulse (normal beat alternating with premature contraction), pulsus bisferiens (double rather than single pulsation)
   c) Abnormalities of quality: hypokinetic (weak) or hyperkinetic (bounding); pulsus alternans (alternation of weak and strong pulses); paradoxical pulse
   d) Thrills palpated or bruits (murmur-like sounds) heard with auscultation

IV. Essential nursing care for client with chest pain

See text pages
_____

A. Nursing assessment
   1. Gather relevant health history information (same as section I of this chapter).
   2. Ask the client to describe the type of pain and its severity; to indicate its location and radiation; and to describe provocative factors, if any (see Nurse Alert, "Assessing Chest Pain").
   3. Ask the client what relieves the pain and what makes it worse.
   4. Assess the client's lifestyle and behavior, including diet, exercise, and responses to stress.
   5. Palpate and auscultate the precordium, listening for normal and abnormal sounds.

B. Nursing diagnoses
   1. Anxiety related to perceived risk of heart attack as expressed by client
   2. Ineffective individual coping related to dysfunctional response to stress as indicated by chest pain

3. Altered nutrition, more than body requirements, related to overconsumption of foods high in saturated fats as revealed by client's weight/height ratio
4. Altered role performance related to perceived risk of heart attack with exertion as indicated by client's low activity levels

---

! N U R S E   *A L E R T* !

Assessing Chest Pain

Use the following information to assess chest pain reported by a client.

Type of Pain	Additional Factors	Possible Cause
Crushing, squeezing, or burning sensation; feeling of heaviness or tightness; dull ache	Triggered by stress, exertion, extreme weather conditions, heavy meals; pain located in substernal area and radiating to left shoulder, arm, jaw, or neck	Angina pectoris, myocardial infarction (MI)
Ripping, tearing pain, throbbing in chest with heartbeat	Triggered by lifting heavy weight or spontaneous; pain located in anterior chest radiating to neck, back, or abdomen	Dissecting aortic aneurysm
Sharp, stabbing pain, knife-like	Triggered by coughing, swallowing, laughing, deep breathing, movement; pain located in substernal region radiating to shoulder, back, or neck	Postmyocardial syndrome, pericarditis

Keep in mind possible non-cardiac causes of chest pain, such as:

- Acute pulmonary embolism
- Esophageal rupture
- Esophageal spasm
- Gastroesophageal reflux (heartburn)
- Musculoskeletal injuries (thoracic)
- Pneumonia
- Pneumothorax
- Rib fracture

5. Altered health maintenance related to knowledge deficit concerning health maintenance behaviors

C. Nursing implementation (intervention)
   1. Educate client concerning possible causes of chest pain and the effectiveness of available therapy.
   2. Educate client concerning appropriate health maintenance activities and possible necessary lifestyle changes, including need for proper diet and exercise.
   3. Help client determine appropriate steps to improve diet and exercise level.

D. Nursing evaluation
   1. Client demonstrates through verbalization an understanding of the importance of a thorough medical evaluation to determine cause of chest pain.
   2. Client demonstrates through verbalization an understanding of the importance of diet and exercise for preventing cardiovascular disease.
   3. Client can identify foods to be avoided.
   4. Client expresses intention to begin regular exercise.

1. Which of the following is the best description of the nurse's focus when obtaining a cardiovascular health history?

   a. The nurse should focus on family history of heart disease and dietary analysis.
   b. The nurse should focus on client risk factors and the signs and symptoms of heart disease.
   c. The nurse should focus on current health status.
   d. The nurse should focus on current health promotion activities.

2. A 42-year-old black male client makes all of the following statements during his discussion with the nurse. Which of these statements indicates the client's need for further education?

   a. "I know that the risk of high blood pressure is greater in blacks so I get my blood pressure checked regularly."
   b. "I exercise for at least 30 minutes 4 or 5 times a week. I don't always have time, but I know it is important."
   c. "My father died from a heart attack at age 51, but it was because he was overweight and he also smoked. I watch my weight closely and I don't smoke."
   d. "My diet isn't always the best, but I do try to watch my intake of fats and sodium. I also try to limit my caffeine intake."

3. A 25-year-old male client complains of mild chest pain. Which of the following is important for the nurse to know in assessing this complaint?

   a. Chest pain can result from many cardiac disorders as well as pulmonary and gastroesophageal disorders.
   b. Chest pain, in the absence of other symptoms, requires no further assessment in an otherwise healthy adult client.
   c. Chest pain that has a cardiovascular origin is always very severe.
   d. Chest pain in a young adult client without a history of a congenital heart defect is of little concern.

4. A mother brings her 4-week-old female infant into the clinic. The mother reports that the infant has gained 4 ounces of weight since birth and is much smaller than her sibling was at this age. Which of the following questions should the nurse ask next to best assess this infant?

   a. "Is there a history of congenital heart disease in your family?"
   b. "Has your infant experienced any growth delay?"
   c. "Does your infant have any difficulty with feedings?"
   d. "Has your infant received all her immunizations?"

5. Which of the following must the nurse keep in mind when beginning a physical assessment of the cardiovascular system?

   a. An inspection of the client's skin, hair, and nails will provide little data.
   b. Inspection and palpation of the precordium is done only in children and thin adults.
   c. The apical impulse should be auscultated in the fifth left intercostal space at the midclavicular line (MCL) in pediatric clients.
   d. The client should be in a supine position with the head of the bed elevated 30°.

6. The nurse is auscultating the heart sounds of a 32-year-old male client. The nurse should:

   a. Auscultate in all 5 areas of the precordium, listening selectively for each cycle component.
   b. Listen for S_1 and S_2 only in the aortic and pulmonic areas.
   c. Auscultate with the stethoscope diaphragm held lightly on the skin for low-pitched sounds.
   d. Auscultate with the client in the following positions: supine, sitting up and leaning forward, right lateral recumbent.

7. While auscultating a 38-year-old female client's heart sounds, the nurse hears a split S_2 in the second and third left intercostal spaces. Which of the following is the best action for the nurse to take?

   a. The nurse should call the physician to inquire about getting an electrocardiogram (ECG) because this is an abnormal finding.
   b. The nurse should ask the client if she has been taking steroidal medications recently.
   c. The nurse should listen to the heart sound again to determine if it disappears on expiration.
   d. The nurse should ask the client if she may be pregnant.

8. The nurse is auscultating the heart sounds of a 29-year-old female client who has been diagnosed with a heart murmur caused by mitral stenosis. Which of the following should the nurse expect to hear on auscultation?

   a. A high-pitched pansystolic murmur at the lower left sternal border and an audible S_3
   b. A low-pitched diastolic murmur in the apical area with an accentuated S_1 and an opening snap
   c. A high-pitched pansystolic murmur heard at the third through the fifth left intercostal spaces with an obscured A_2
   d. A high-pitched diastolic murmur heard at the second through the fourth left intercostal spaces and an ejection sound

9. The nurse is palpating the arterial pulses of a 34-year-old female client. Which of the following is the correct procedure to follow?

   a. The nurse should press gently on all pulse sites and palpate only 1 carotid artery at a time.
   b. The nurse should avoid palpating arteries that lie over bones.
   c. The nurse should assess the carotid and femoral pulses first. If these are normal, he/she does not need to assess the remaining pulses.

   d. After assessing rate and rhythm, the nurse should attempt to obliterate the pulse at each site.

10. A 56-year-old male client presents to the emergency room with a complaint of chest pain. Which of the following questions would best help the nurse assess whether the client is experiencing angina pectoris or a myocardial infarction (MI)?

    a. "What were you doing when the pain began?"
    b. "Can you describe what the pain is like?"
    c. "Where do you feel the pain?"
    d. "How long have you been in pain?"

11. The nurse has been assigned to care for a 60-year-old woman admitted for the evaluation of chest pain. She admits to the nurse that she is frightened about having chest pain and that she is afraid to die. Which of the following would be the most appropriate nursing diagnosis for this client?

    a. Ineffective individual coping related to need for lifestyle changes secondary to chest pain
    b. High risk for impaired social interaction related to fear of chest pain
    c. Anxiety related to perceived risk of heart attack as expressed by client
    d. Alteration in nutritional intake related to knowledge deficit concerning heart disease risk factors

12. The nurse is performing an assessment of a 65-year-old male client who entered the hospital after an MI. He has recently been moved out of the coronary care unit to another floor. He will be discharged to home care within 72 hours if his progress continues. Which of the following points is the best one for the nurse to emphasize to facilitate client education?

    a. Teach the client how to assess his peripheral pulses and record them on a daily basis.
    b. Teach the client about the need for a low-fat, high-fiber diet and regular, appropriate exercise.

c. Teach the client about the need to have his blood pressure checked weekly.

d. Teach the client about the necessity for keeping his monthly ECG appointments.

ANSWERS

1. **Correct answer is b.** The complete cardiovascular health history must include an assessment of the client's signs and symptoms of heart disease and must also include an evaluation of cardiovascular risk factors. The signs and symptoms of some cardiovascular diseases take years to manifest themselves, and knowledge about a client's risk factors can help focus the assessment.

   a. Information about family history of heart disease and dietary intake are generally included in the assessment of cardiovascular risk factors.
   c. Focusing only on the client's current health status may not provide the information needed.
   d. Health promotion is generally included in the assessment of the cardiovascular risk factors.

2. **Correct answer is c.** The client doesn't understand the role of heredity as a risk factor for developing heart disease. Cardiac disease before the age of 55 in a blood relative increases a client's risk.

   a, b, and **d.** These statements all reflect an understanding of cardiovascular risk factors and appropriate client response.

3. **Correct answer is a.** Chest pain can result from a variety of causes, including pulmonary and gastroesophageal as well as cardiac. A careful study of signs and symptoms and a thorough assessment is needed.

   b. Chest pain may be of little concern in an otherwise healthy adult, but it should always be evaluated.
   c. Chest pain of cardiac origin is not always severe; the pain of angina pectoris, for example, is sometimes mistaken for indigestion.

d. Although certain kinds of heart disorders are rare in young adults without heart defects, chest pain is always a cause for concern. Also, an individual may have an undiagnosed but serious heart defect.

4. **Correct answer is c.** Children with congestive heart failure (CHF) or congenital heart disease may have difficulty with feedings because their hearts cannot provide the additional energy needed for the feeding process.

   a. While a family history of congenital heart disease may be of interest as the nurse gathers data about this infant, it is not the best question to ask next.
   b. The mother has already answered this question by the only measure she has— weight gain. The nurse needs to ask a different question.
   d. Immunization information is not essential for diagnosis of a heart problem.

5. **Correct answer is d.** This is a description of the optimal client position. Proper positioning is essential for the collection of accurate data.

   a. A general inspection of the skin and nails can provide useful information about circulatory function.
   b. Inspection and palpation provide very useful information for all clients.
   c. Although this is the usual position for adult clients, the apical impulse is higher in children under 7.

6. **Correct answer is a.** To assess heart sounds thoroughly, the nurse must always auscultate in all 5 areas of the precordium. By singling out each individual heart component the nurse can carefully note any abnormalities such as extra sounds or splitting in each area.

   b. S_1 and S_2 should be listened for in each of the 5 precordial areas. S_1 is often louder at the apex and lower sternal border and S_2 is often louder at the base.
   c. This is an incorrect description of how to use the stethoscope. The diaphragm is held firmly on the skin and is best used for hearing high-pitched sounds.

d. This is an incorrect description of client positions. The heart should be auscultated with the client supine, sitting up and leaning forward, and left lateral recumbent.

7. **Correct answer is c.** A split S_2 is normal on inspiration in adults but should disappear on expiration. A split S_2 may occur normally during both inspiration and expiration in children.

   a. The nurse should assess further to determine whether this is an abnormal finding before asking a physician to order any diagnostic tests.
   b. Use of steroidal medications may have effects on the cardiovascular system but would not result in this finding.
   d. This finding is not one normally associated with pregnancy; findings normally associated with pregnancy include certain types of murmurs and a slight displacement of the heart.

8. **Correct answer is b.** The murmur caused by mitral stenosis is heard in mid- to late diastole at the apex of the heart. The pitch is low (the nurse should use the stethoscope bell for auscultation) and an accentuated S_1 is often present along with an opening snap that follows S_2. Mitral regurgitation may also occur.

   a. These findings are indicative of a murmur caused by tricuspid regurgitation.
   c. These findings are indicative of a murmur caused by a ventricular septal defect.
   d. These findings are indicative of a murmur caused by aortic regurgitation.

9. **Correct answer is a.** Pressing gently on the pulse sites will help the nurse avoid obliterating the pulse and thereby obtaining a false reading. The nurse should avoid palpating both carotid arteries at the same time because doing so can decrease the blood supply to the brain.

   b. All the pulse sites are in areas where the arteries lie over bone, making them easier to palpate.
   c. The nurse should always assess all pulse sites. Normal carotid and femoral pulses do not suggest normal readings for any other pulse site.

d. The nurse does not need to obliterate the pulse at any site, although he/she will assess the strength of the pulse. Obliterating the pulse in some sites could compromise circulation for the client.

10. **Correct answer is d.** The duration of pain is one of the ways to differentiate chest pain associated with angina from that of an MI. The pain associated with angina tends to last for 5–10 minutes at a time, building and then fading. The pain of an MI is constant.

    a. The provocative factors for the 2 conditions are very similar. This question would not help the nurse distinguish the etiology.
    b. Both types of pain are often described as crushing or squeezing or as a feeling of heaviness or pressure.
    c. Both types of pain are felt in the substernal region and may radiate to the left shoulder, jaw, or arm.

11. **Correct answer is c.** The client is expressing her fears about having another attack of chest pain.

    a. The nurse does not have enough data about her coping skills to make this diagnosis. Also, the client has not expressed difficulty in coping with lifestyle changes.
    b. Nothing expressed by the client implies that her fears about another attack are adversely affecting her social interactions.
    d. Nothing stated by the client reveals an alteration in nutrition related to a knowledge deficit in this area.

12. **Correct answer is b.** The client needs to understand the diet and exercise requirements for improved cardiac health.

    a. Assessing and recording peripheral pulses daily will not be part of the home care plan for this client.
    c. Although weekly blood pressure readings are a good idea, they will not be part of the client's home care plan.
    d. The client will not be required to have monthly ECGs. An occasional ECG will be scheduled.

8

The Breasts and Axillae

OVERVIEW

I. **Relevant health history**
   A. Current status
   B. Past status
   C. Family history
   D. Risk factors: breast cancer
   E. Developmental
      considerations

II. **Anatomy and physiology**
   A. Male breast
   B. Female breast
   C. Lymphatic system

III. **Assessment techniques**
   A. Inspection and palpation of
      the male breast and axilla
   B. Inspection and palpation of
      the female breast and axilla

IV. **Special diagnostic
   techniques**
   A. Mammography
   B. Xerography
   C. Transillumination
   D. Biopsy

V. **Essential nursing care for
   female client reporting
   detection of a breast lump**
   A. Nursing assessment
   B. Nursing diagnoses
   C. Nursing implementation
      (intervention)
   D. Nursing evaluation

NURSING HIGHLIGHTS

1. Breast cancer is the second leading cause of death among women, so thorough examinations and client education are vital.
2. Approximately 70%–80% of lesions detected through breast-cancer screening are benign, a fact to be emphasized during client education.
3. Examination of a male's breasts can usually be brief, but carefully checking the lymph nodes is important; 1%–5% of breast cancers occur in males.
4. Some women may be uncomfortable during examination of the breasts, so courtesy, gentleness, warm hands, privacy, and a matter-of-fact approach are important.

5. The nurse must be sensitive to the fact that in the United States, female breasts are associated with sexuality; consequently the threat of a potentially disfiguring disease such as breast cancer can greatly affect the woman's body image, feelings of personal worth, and relationships with others.

GLOSSARY

acini—small saclike glandular structures in the female breasts that produce milk

gynecomastia—a condition characterized by abnormal growth of breast tissue among males

Paget's disease—cancer of the breast characterized by scaling around the nipple and usually accompanied by a malignancy deeper in the breast

peau d'orange—dimpled appearance of skin resembling the skin of an orange; condition caused by edema; usually associated with underlying disease

striae—pink or purple lines seen on the breasts that turn lighter over time; condition results from rapid increase in skin tension

ENHANCED OUTLINE

I. Relevant health history

A. Current status
  1. Does the client notice any changes in the breasts or axillae?
     a) Description (e.g., presence of masses or swelling, changes in pigmentation, presence of rash or eczema on the nipple, evidence of tenderness, observation of nipple discharge)
     b) Cause: Some changes are variations that occur normally during the menstrual cycle or as a result of certain medications; others may be indicative of disease.
  2. Does the client regularly examine his/her own breasts?

B. Past status
  1. Has client noted changes in the breasts or axillae in the past?
  2. What was the age of onset of menarche/menopause?
  3. Has the client had breast surgery? If so, for what reason?
  4. Has the client borne any children? If so, at what age(s)?
  5. What is the client's breastfeeding history?
  6. Did the client experience excessive weight gain after onset of menopause?
  7. Has the client had regular mammograms, as recommended for her age?

C. Family history: Has a mother or sister been diagnosed with breast cancer?

> See text pages
> _____

D. Risk factors: breast cancer
1. Family history of breast cancer (mother or sister, especially premenopausally)
2. Age: 80% of breast cancers occur in women older than 40
3. Previous cancer in 1 breast
4. Early menarche (before age 12): Breasts are exposed to increased levels of estrogen for a longer period.
5. Late menopause (after age 55): Breasts are exposed to increased levels of estrogen for a longer period.
6. Late or no pregnancies: Bearing no children or bearing the first child after age 30 increases risk.
7. Previous exposure to excessive ionizing radiation, as with frequent chest x-rays
8. Others, including high dietary intake of fat, cystic breast disease with epithelial hyperplasia, prior use of estrogen or androgens to suppress lactation

E. Developmental considerations
1. Age-related changes
   a) Puberty: Development of adult breasts begins.
      (1) Stage 1: Nipple elevation begins.
      (2) Stage 2: Breast buds appear.
      (3) Stage 3: Breasts and areolae grow.
      (4) Stage 4: Secondary mounds form.
      (5) Stage 5: Breasts take on adult contours.
   b) Menopause: Glandular tissue disappears; breasts become flat and flaccid.
2. Pregnancy-related changes
   a) Breasts increase in size.
   b) Areolae and nipples increase in size and become more darkly pigmented.
   c) Veins become more prominent.
   d) Striae can develop.
3. Breastfeeding-related changes
   a) Breasts can become engorged.
   b) Nipples can become irritated.

II. Anatomy and physiology

See text pages
_____

A. Male breast
1. Made up of nipple, areola, lymphatic system, and breast tissue
2. Usually not palpably distinguishable from the surrounding tissue

B. Female breast
   1. Milk-producing structures
      a) Each breast made up of 15–25 lobes.
      b) Each lobe made up of 20–40 lobules.
      c) Each lobule made up of 10–100 acini.
   2. Fat tissue: surrounds glandular lobes
   3. External structures: nipple, areola, Montgomery's tubercle
   4. Supporting structures: subcutaneous connective tissue, Cooper's ligament (suspensory), pectoral muscle

C. Lymphatic system: network of tissues that defend against microorganism invasion and carry malignant cells away from neoplasms
   1. A separate system drains lymph from each breast, returning it to the blood.
   2. Cancer can spread through the lymphatic system to the other breast or to some more distant location such as the abdomen.
      a) Pectoral (anterior) lymph nodes
         (1) Located on the lower edge of the pectoralis major muscle and inside the anterior fold of the axilla
         (2) Drain most of the breast and the anterior chest wall
      b) Brachial (lateral) lymph nodes
         (1) Located at the upper end of the humerus
         (2) Drain most of the arm

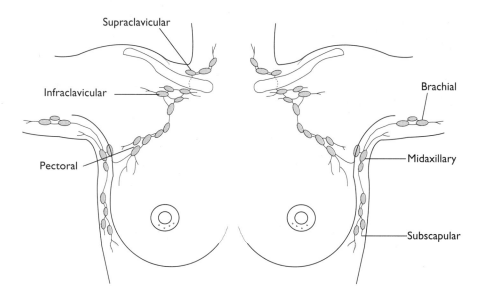

Figure 8–1
Location of Lymph Nodes

        c) Subscapular (posterior) lymph nodes
          (1) Located along the lateral border of the scapula, deep within the posterior fold of the axilla
          (2) Drain part of the arm and the posterior chest wall
        d) Midaxillary (central) lymph nodes
          (1) Located deep within the axilla, close to the ribs and the serratus anterior muscle
          (2) Drain lymph from the pectoral, brachial, and subscapular lymph nodes
        e) Supraclavicular and infraclavicular lymph nodes
          (1) Located above (supraclavicular) and below (infraclavicular) the clavicle
          (2) Drain lymph from the midaxillary lymph nodes and deep breast tissues

III. Assessment techniques

> See text pages
> _____

A. Inspection and palpation of the male breast and axilla
    1. Inspection: The various positions used when examining a female client's breast are not necessary when examining a male client.
        a) With client in sitting position, inspect the nipple and areola for masses, swelling, or sores.
        b) Inspect the skin of the axilla for increased pigmentation, rash, or infection.
    2. Palpation
        a) With client in supine position, palpate the areola and nipple for nodules and the breast tissue for gynecomastia.
        b) With client in sitting position, palpate the lymph nodes of the axilla.
          (1) Midaxillary lymph nodes: Push the fingertips as high into the axilla as they will go, press them against the chest wall, and slide them downward to feel the nodes.
          (2) Pectoral lymph nodes: Grasp the anterior axillary fold with the thumb and fingers to feel the nodes.
          (3) Brachial lymph nodes: Press the fingers high into the axilla and feel the nodes against the end of the humerus.
          (4) Subscapular lymph nodes: From behind the client, grasp the posterior axillary fold inside the muscle to feel the nodes.
          (5) Supraclavicular lymph nodes: Flex client's head forward slightly and hook index finger over clavicle; press fingers inward to feel nodes.
          (6) Infraclavicular lymph nodes: same as section III,A,2,b,1 of this chapter

B. Inspection and palpation of the female breast and axilla
   1. Inspection
      a) With the client in a sitting position, check skin for irregularities.
         (1) Unusual color changes can indicate underlying infection or inflammatory carcinoma.
         (2) Thickening, prominent pores and veins, dimpling, retractions, or peau d'orange can indicate underlying cancer.
      b) Check the breasts, areolae, and nipples for symmetry of size, shape, and placement.
         (1) Breasts should be symmetrical in size and shape; a slight difference in size between the breasts is normal.
         (2) Flattening of the curve of the breast, a recently retracted nipple, or deviation of the directions in which the nipples point can indicate underlying cancer.
      c) Check the areolae and nipples for rash, ulceration, or discharge.
         (1) Rash or ulceration can indicate Paget's disease.
         (2) Discharge can indicate presence of cancer.
      d) Check the axillae for unusual pigmentation or swelling.
         (1) Increased pigmentation can indicate cancer.
         (2) Swelling can indicate infection or cancer.
      e) Have client use alternative positions to check the breasts for symmetry of size, shape, and placement.
         (1) With the client at rest with arms at sides
         (2) As client raises arms over head
         (3) With the client sitting straight with hands pressed against hips
         (4) With the client leaning forward

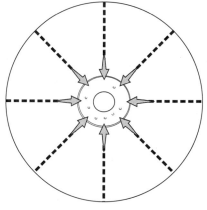

Palpate in wedge sections from periphery to center

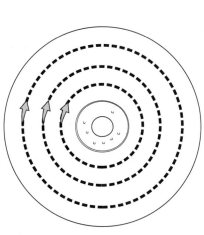

Palpate in concentric circles

Figure 8–2
Systematic Palpation Techniques

2. Palpation
   a) Breast
      (1) Use the same systematic pattern of palpation with each breast examination.
         (a) Wedge sections (palpated like the spokes of a wheel)
         (b) Concentric circles
      (2) Use 2 client positions when examining the breast.
         (a) With the client in a supine position, place a pillow under the shoulder of the breast to be examined (unless the breasts are small) and palpate with 1 hand.
         (b) With the client in a sitting position, palpate with both hands.
      (3) Examine the entire area using the finger pads, from the clavicle to below the inframammary fold and from the midsternal line to the posterior axillary fold, paying special attention to the upper outer quadrant and the tail of Spence (half of all cancers occur here).
      (4) Check the breast, areola, and axilla for consistency of tissue, tenderness, masses.
      (5) Describe any mass detected.
         (a) Its location using clock or quadrant reference and distance from nipple in centimeters
         (b) Its size in centimeters
         (c) Its shape: round or discoid; regular or irregular
         (d) Its consistency: soft or hard; cystic or solid
         (e) If it is discrete
         (f) If it is mobile or fixed to underlying tissue
         (g) If it is tender
         (h) If skin dimpling is present
      (6) Compress nipple between thumb and index finger and describe any discharge.
         (a) The lobe from which it originates
         (b) Its color: milky or nonmilky
      (7) Make a cytologic smear of abnormal discharge.
   b) Axilla (same as section III,A,2,b of this chapter)

IV. Special diagnostic techniques

See text pages
_____

A. Mammography: low-energy radiographic technique that reveals internal lesions

B. Xerography: radiographic technique similar to mammography, but using lower doses of radiation and yielding crisper images

C. Transillumination: diagnostic technique involving the use of infrared light to see through breast tissue; data transformed by computer into images of light (normal tissue) and dark (lesions)

D. Biopsy: definitive diagnostic procedure involving the removal of a sample of the lesion for examination

V. Essential nursing care for female client reporting detection of a breast lump

See text pages
_____

A. Nursing assessment
  1. Gather relevant health history information (same as section I of this chapter).
  2. Ask the client to point to the area where the lump was detected and to demonstrate the method that led to the detection of the lump.
  3. Inspect the breast for abnormalities: flattening of the breast's shape; thickening of the skin; prominent pores and veins; dimpling;

✔ CLIENT TEACHING CHECKLIST ✔

Performing a Breast Self-Examination

Explain the following breast self-examination steps to the client:

✔ Have the client disrobe to the waist and stand in front of a mirror with her arms at her sides.

✔ Have the client observe for abnormalities at rest with arms at sides and again as she raises her arms slowly, as she presses her hands against her hips and flexes her pectoral muscles, and as she bends forward at the waist (large-breasted women only).

— Dimpling

— Retraction or deviation of the nipples

— Flattening of the breast curve

— Peau d'orange

✔ Demonstrate systematic, thorough palpation by guiding the client's hand during palpation of the breast.

✔ Instruct the client to perform a thorough palpation while standing (many individuals prefer to a do a breast self-examination in the shower because the soap and water help the hands glide more easily over the skin) and again while lying down with a pillow placed under the shoulder of the side being examined.

✔ Have the client squeeze the nipple and observe for discharge.

---

retractions; peau d'orange; recent nipple deviation, retraction, or discharge; rash, ulceration, or change in pigmentation of the skin of the breast, areolae, nipples, or axillae.

4. Palpate the breast to determine if lumps or other abnormalities are present.
5. Thoroughly assess any masses detected (same as section III,B,2,a,5 of this chapter).
6. Assess client's knowledge of normal female physiology, breast cancer risk factors, and breast self-examination techniques.

B. Nursing diagnoses
   1. Anxiety related to perceived potential for breast cancer as expressed by client
   2. Anxiety related to knowledge deficit concerning normal female physiology
   3. Altered health maintenance related to knowledge deficit concerning breast cancer risk factors
   4. Noncompliance related to knowledge deficit concerning breast self-examination techniques

C. Nursing implementation (intervention)
   1. Educate client regarding breast physiology and cancer risk factors.
   2. Explain to client normal breast changes (such as those occurring during menstruation) and those that may be abnormal.
   3. Teach the client how to examine her own breasts (see Client Teaching Checklist, "Performing a Breast Self-Examination").

D. Nursing evaluation
   1. Client demonstrates through verbalization an understanding of breast physiology and is aware of cancer risk factors.
   2. Client demonstrates through verbalization an understanding of normal breast changes and those that may be abnormal.
   3. Client is able to examine her breasts using correct techniques.

1. Many women avoid breast exams and mammograms because:

   a. Data are inconclusive concerning their effectiveness in the early detection of breast cancer.

   b. Most women perform a breast self-examination every month.

   c. Breast cancer is a relatively uncommon disease.

   d. The breasts are closely linked to a woman's body image and sexuality.

2. A 43-year-old female client has never had a mammogram. During the health history, she reluctantly tells the nurse that her maternal aunt died from breast cancer and that her sister, age 38, had a lumpectomy last year for a malignant growth. The best nursing action is to:

   a. Schedule a mammogram for her immediately.

   b. Share with her the risk factors for breast cancer.

   c. Explore her concerns about breast cancer and mammograms.

   d. Ask if she has ever been pregnant or breastfed any of her children.

3. Which of the following breast changes are considered normal during the course of pregnancy?

   a. Pendulous breasts with nipples pointing downward

   b. Right breast slightly larger than left, pink areolae

   c. Dark areolae, enlarged breasts, and appearance of striae

   d. Swollen areolae and developing breast buds

4. A woman who has had breast cancer in 1 breast has an increased risk of developing cancer in her other breast. One reason for this may be that:

   a. Both breasts have similar fatty tissue, and therefore both are susceptible to cancer.

   b. Cancer cells from 1 breast may cross to the other breast via the lymphatic system.

   c. Breastfeeding causes changes in both breasts.

   d. Cancer in another body area may spread to the breasts via the milk line.

5. When assessing the breast and axillae, particular attention should be paid to the brachial nodes. To palpate the brachial nodes, the following technique is correct:

   a. Press the pads of the fingers of both hands deeply into the axilla until the ribs are felt.

   b. Grasp the tail of Spence between the thumb and fingers and palpate the tissue.

   c. With the pads of the fingers, palpate the breast in a concentric pattern.

   d. Using the pads of the fingers of both hands, try to compress the nodes against the upper inner aspect of the humerus.

6. The nurse is performing a breast exam and asks the client to flex her head forward while the nurse hooks her own fingers over the client's clavicle and presses inward. Which group of lymph nodes is the nurse assessing?

   a. Supraclavicular

   b. Subscapular

   c. Midaxillary

   d. Inguinal

7. Which of the following assessment findings is normal?

   a. Firm inframammary ridge

   b. Skin dimpling in lower outer quadrant

   c. Unequal nipple axis

   d. Peau d'orange skin above the areola

8. Most malignant breast lumps in women are found in the:

   a. Upper inner quadrant.
   b. Left inner quadrant.
   c. Axilla.
   d. Upper outer quadrant.

9. Which of the following techniques is recommended in assessment of the breast and axilla?

   a. Using a cupped palm, palpate each breast in concentric circles or wedge sections.
   b. When the client is in a sitting position, inspect the breasts as she crosses her arms.
   c. Use bimanual palpation of large, pendulous breasts while the client is sitting.
   d. Using the tip of the index finger, press into the breast in all quadrants and in the areola.

10. A nurse in a certified breast center sees a 57-year-old female client who requests an exam and a mammogram. Palpation of her left breast reveals a nontender 2×2×3 cm mass in the upper outer quadrant that is rock-hard, immobile, and has an irregular border. The client never performs breast self-exams, so she has never noticed the lump. This mass displays the characteristics of a(n):

    a. Calcified milk duct.
    b. Tumor, possibly malignant.
    c. Fluid-filled cyst.
    d. Enlarged, inflamed lymph node.

11. The nurse is completing a health history with a new client. The 45-year-old female client tells the nurse that she had a right mastectomy for breast cancer when she was 32 years old. She performs a breast self-exam every month and has always kept her follow-up appointments for exams and mammograms. She states she should be happy that the cancer has never recurred; however, she can't help feeling embarrassed and ashamed of her body. She has never married and is now dating a man who knows nothing of her breast cancer or mastectomy. She asks the nurse about breast reconstructive surgery. The most appropriate nursing diagnosis for her is:

    a. Altered health maintenance related to ineffective coping.
    b. Self-esteem disturbance related to high risk for physical deformity.
    c. Anxiety related to knowledge deficit concerning breast cancer recurrence rates.
    d. Body image disturbance related to perception of physical deformity.

12. Which of the following nursing actions would most effectively increase the early detection rate of breast cancer in women over age 50?

    a. Recommending yearly chest x-rays to all female clients
    b. Teaching clients by distributing pamphlets on breast cancer risk factors
    c. Motivating clients to perform a breast self-exam every 3 months and a baseline mammogram before the age of 45
    d. Teaching clients to perform a monthly breast self-exam and to obtain a yearly mammogram and exam by a health professional

ANSWERS

1. **Correct answer is d.** Many women are uncomfortable about having other persons, even if they are health professionals, touch their breasts.

   a. Mammograms and breast exams have proven to be very effective in the early detection of breast cancer.
   b. Most women do not perform a breast self-examination every month.
   c. Breast cancer is the second leading cause of death among women. One in 9 women will develop breast cancer.

2. **Correct answer is c.** The client's concerns about breast cancer and available methods of early detection take priority at this time.

 a. The client definitely needs a mammogram, but she may not comply unless her concerns are addressed first.

 b. This client does have some risk factors for breast cancer, but going over them at this time is likely to increase her anxiety.

 d. You will want to know this later, but it is not an appropriate question at this time.

3. **Correct answer is c.** Enlarged breasts with darkened areolae and striae are all common breast changes during pregnancy.

 a. Pendulous breasts with downward pointing nipples are common breast changes in the elderly female population.

 b. Having pink areolae and 1 breast slightly larger than the other are normal findings in the nulliparous adult woman.

 d. The development of breast buds and puffy areolae are normal findings in pubescent girls.

4. **Correct answer is b.** The lymphatic system connects both breasts and may convey cancer cells from 1 to the other. Cancer cells may also travel from the breasts to the abdomen.

 a. The similarity of fatty breast tissue does not *increase* the risk of developing breast cancer in both breasts.

 c. Breastfeeding does cause breast changes, but it also offers some protection against breast cancer.

 d. The milk line is on the outer surface of the skin, from the axilla to the groin. Supernumerary nipples or breast tissue may form along this line, but there is no channel to spread cancer cells.

5. **Correct answer is d.** This is the proper technique for palpating the brachial nodes, which are located in the upper inner aspect of the arm.

 a. This is part of the technique to feel the midaxillary lymph nodes.

 b. This is part of the technique to feel the pectoral lymph nodes.

 c. This is a correct technique for palpating breast tissue.

6. **Correct answer is a.** The supraclavicular nodes lie close to the chest wall above the clavicle.

 b. The subscapular nodes are palpated by grasping the posterior axillary fold from behind the client.

 c. The midaxillary nodes are palpated by pushing the fingers high into the axilla, pressing against the chest wall, and then sliding them downward.

 d. The inguinal nodes are palpated in the groin area and are not usually associated with the lymph nodes of the breast.

7. **Correct answer is a.** A firm ridge of tissue can be felt as a half circle under the breasts. This is the inframammary ridge, a normal finding.

 b. Dimpling, along with retraction of skin, is usually caused by the shortening of Cooper's ligament by an invasive mass.

 c. When inspecting the breasts, an imaginary horizontal line drawn through the nipples should be parallel to the floor. If 1 nipple is visibly higher or lower or is pointing in a different direction, an underlying tumor may be present.

 d. Roughened, thickened, orange-peel-like skin is a sign of lymphatic blockage, usually a result of malignancy.

8. **Correct answer is d.** Over 50% of malignant breast masses are found in the upper outer quadrant, including the tail of Spence.

 a, b, and **c.** Malignant breast lumps may be found in these areas, but the majority are not.

9. **Correct answer is c.** If the breasts are large, compressing a lump between 2 hands may be the only way to find it. Otherwise the lump may slide into deeper tissues.

 a. The fingerpads, not cupped palms, are used to palpate each breast in concentric circles or wedge sections.

b. When the client is in a sitting position, inspect the breasts as she raises her arms and places her hands on her hips.
d. This may cause discomfort and will yield no useful assessment data.

10. **Correct answer is b.** A malignant tumor can be definitively diagnosed only with a biopsy, but this mass displays many characteristics common to malignant tumors.

    a. A calcified milk duct is very firm, usually smooth, and located under the areola.
    c. A fluid-filled cyst does not feel rock-hard and usually has a smooth, regular border.
    d. An enlarged, inflamed lymph node is very tender and may be painful on palpation.

11. **Correct answer is d.** She does not feel comfortable with her body in its current state and is thinking about changing it.

    a. She has been maintaining her health related to preventing breast cancer by recommended methods.

b. Although she may have a self-esteem disturbance, her deformity has already occurred.
c. No data are given that support a knowledge deficit on breast cancer rates.

12. **Correct answer is d.** This is part of the currently recommended guidelines for breast screening of women without signs and symptoms of breast disease.

    a. Having yearly chest x-rays increases a client's exposure to radiation and is not recommended for the detection of breast cancer.
    b. Distributing pamphlets, although helpful, is not a substitute for one-on-one teaching. Knowledge of cancer risk factors is useless unless the client is taught the best methods to detect cancer early: breast self-exams and regular mammograms.
    c. Clients should be taught to perform a breast self-exam *every* month. The baseline mammogram should be obtained before the age of 40.

9

The Abdomen

OVERVIEW

I. Relevant health history
  A. Current status
  B. Past status
  C. Family history

II. Anatomy and physiology
  A. Abdominal landmarks
  B. Major abdominal organs

III. Assessment techniques
  A. Approach
  B. Inspection

C. Auscultation
D. Percussion
E. Palpation

IV. Essential nursing care for client with abdominal pain
  A. Nursing assessment
  B. Nursing diagnoses
  C. Nursing implementation (intervention)
  D. Nursing evaluation

NURSING HIGHLIGHTS

1. Many clients are embarrassed to discuss gastrointestinal (GI) function, especially elimination. Privacy is important throughout the assessment.
2. Remember the 6 "F's" that are the common causes of abdominal distention: fluid, fat, flatulence, feces, fibroid tumor, and fetus.
3. Auscultation of the abdomen normally precedes percussion and palpation because percussion and palpation can stimulate bowel motility and increase the frequency of bowel sounds.

GLOSSARY

ascites—an abnormal accumulation of fluid in the peritoneal cavity
bruit—a murmur-like sound heard over blood vessels
peristalsis—waves of involuntary contractions in a muscular tube of the body (e.g., the intestines, ureters)

I. Relevant health history

See text pages
_____

A. Current status
1. Does the client have pain in the stomach or abdomen?
   a) Description (e.g., sharp, dull, knife-like, cramping)
   b) Location and radiation
   c) Onset, frequency, and timing of episodes
   d) Palliative or provocative factors (e.g., food, antacids, alcohol, movement, rest)
   e) Treatments
2. Is the client experiencing nausea and/or vomiting?
   a) Frequency and timing of episodes
   b) Characteristics of vomitus (e.g, color, blood, odor)
3. Is the client's abdomen swollen?
4. Is the client experiencing constipation or diarrhea?
5. Does the client frequently use laxatives or enemas?
   a) Reason for and frequency of use
   b) Type or brand used
6. What over-the-counter (OTC) and prescription medications is the client taking and for what conditions?

B. Past status
1. Has the client experienced a change in diet or eating habits?
   a) Description (e.g., change in appetite, weight loss or gain)
   b) Onset (approximate date, gradual or sudden)
2. Has the client experienced a change in urination or bowel habits?
3. Has the client had abdominal surgery?
   a) Date and type of surgery
   b) Residual effects
4. Has the client been diagnosed with any food allergies?
5. Has the client had previous problems with liver or kidney disease, colitis, peptic ulcers, or cancer of any abdominal organ?

C. Family history: Has anyone in the client's family been diagnosed with liver or kidney disease, colorectal cancer, colitis, or peptic ulcer?

II. Anatomy and physiology

See text pages
_____

A. Abdominal landmarks: 2 methods for locating abdominal structures
1. The 4 quadrants: created by 2 imaginary perpendicular lines crossing at umbilicus
   a) Right upper quadrant (RUQ): majority of liver, gallbladder, pylorus, duodenum, head of pancreas, right adrenal gland, portion

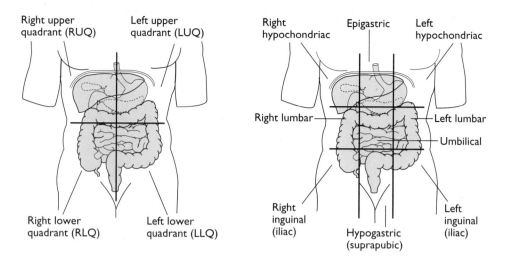

Figure 9–1
Abdominal Landmarks

of right kidney, hepatic flexure of colon, portions of ascending and transverse colon

   b) Right lower quadrant (RLQ): cecum, appendix, portion of ascending colon, lowest pole of right kidney, right ureter, right ovary and salpinx or right spermatic cord

   c) Left upper quadrant (LUQ): stomach, left liver lobe, spleen, body of pancreas, left adrenal gland, left kidney, splenic flexure of colon, portions of transverse and descending colon

   d) Left lower quadrant (LLQ): sigmoid colon, portion of descending colon, left ureter, left ovary and salpinx or left spermatic cord

2. The 9 regions

   a) Created by 2 imaginary vertical lines extending from midclavicles through middle of inguinal ligament and 2 imaginary horizontal lines at costal margin and iliac crests

   b) Regions: right hypochondriac, right lumbar, right inguinal (iliac), epigastric, umbilical, hypogastric (suprapubic), left hypochondriac, left lumbar, left inguinal (iliac)

B. Major abdominal organs

   1. Stomach

      a) J-shaped pouch located beneath diaphragm

      b) 3 sections: fundus, body or corpus, and pylorus

      c) 2 sphincters controlling flow in and out of stomach: cardiac sphincter (from esophagus) and pyloric sphincter (to duodenum)

      d) Major functions: storage and breakdown of food into chyme

   2. Small intestine

      a) Long coiled tube (6.4 m) located in central and lower portion of abdomen; opens into large intestine

b) 3 sections: duodenum, jejunum, and ileum
c) Major functions: digestion and absorption of nutrients
3. Large intestine
   a) Tube (1.5 m) extending from small intestine to anus
   b) 3 sections: cecum (with vermiform appendix); colon (ascending colon, transverse colon, descending colon, sigmoid colon); and rectum
   c) Major functions: completion of absorption; formation and expulsion of feces
4. Liver
   a) Large gland located in RUQ and LUQ beneath diaphragm
   b) Right lobe and left lobe; right lobe further divided into caudate lobe and quadrate lobe
   c) Major functions: production and secretion of bile, storage of various vitamins and minerals, metabolism, and detoxification
5. Gallbladder
   a) Small pear-shaped organ located under right lobe of liver
   b) Major functions: storage and concentration of bile
6. Pancreas
   a) Narrow, oblong organ lying behind the stomach
   b) Divided into 3 sections: head, body, and tail
   c) Major functions
      (1) Exocrine: secretion of enzymes to aid digestion in small intestine
      (2) Endocrine: secretion of hormones to regulate glucose levels
7. Spleen
   a) Large lymphoid organ located in LUQ between diaphragm and stomach
   b) 2 tissue types: red pulp and white pulp
   c) Major functions: immunologic functions such as replacement of worn-out blood cells and removal of bacteria; storage of blood
8. Kidneys, ureters, and bladder
   a) Location
      (1) Kidneys: paired, bean-shaped organs located in dorsal abdomen between 12th thoracic and third lumbar vertebrae; right kidney slightly lower than left
      (2) Ureters: tubes that drain kidneys; pass anteriorly along psoas major muscles into bladder
      (3) Bladder: spherical organ behind symphysis pubis; rises above symphysis pubis when distended
   b) Containing more than 1 million nephrons (functional units), each composed of glomerulus and tubular system

    c) Major functions
       (1) Kidneys: production of urine, filtration of wastes, and reabsorption of substances needed by the body
       (2) Ureters: transportation of urine to bladder
       (3) Bladder: storage of urine until elimination
9. Peritoneum
    a) Serous membrane surrounding organs of the abdominal cavity
    b) 2 layers, parietal and visceral, and 2 folds, mesentery and omentum (greater and lesser)
    c) Major functions: binds organs to each other and to abdominal cavity walls, supplies blood and nerves to abdominal organs

III. Assessment techniques

See text pages
_____

A. Approach
  1. Room temperature should be comfortable; examiner's hands and stethoscope should be warmed.
  2. Client should be relaxed and supine with arms at sides or folded over chest; small pillow beneath head and knees may aid comfort.
  3. Client's bladder should be empty.
  4. Abdomen should be fully exposed from above xiphoid process to symphysis pubis; genitalia and chest should be draped.

B. Inspection
  1. With single source of light (overhead or tangential), inspect from right side at abdomen level; inspect again standing at foot of table and when client takes a deep breath.
  2. Inspect shape of abdomen for symmetry and contour (flat, round, scaphoid, or distended); note any masses.
  3. Inspect skin for pigmentation (particularly signs of jaundice), lesions, striae, dilated veins, and scars.
  4. Inspect umbilicus, noting contour and location as well as any signs of inflammation or umbilical hernia (bulging).
  5. Inspect for visible signs of peristalsis; visible waves may indicate intestinal obstruction.
  6. Inspect for pulsations; epigastric aortic pulsations may be normal.
  7. Ask client to raise head and shoulders; inspect abdomen for hernia.

C. Auscultation
  1. Bowel (peristaltic) sounds
    a) Lightly press diaphragm of stethoscope on abdomen; note character and frequency of bowel sounds.
    b) Note normal findings.
       (1) Soft clicks and gurgles normally occur 5–34 times per minute.
       (2) Borborygmi (prolonged gurgles or stomach growling) may be normal if client is hungry.
    c) Document abnormal findings.
       (1) Increased bowel sounds may indicate diarrhea or early intestinal obstruction.

(2) Markedly decreased or absent bowel sounds may indicate peritonitis, late bowel obstruction, or paralytic ileus; auscultate again after several minutes.

2. Vascular sounds
   a) Listen for bruits with bell and diaphragm over arteries.
      (1) Aorta
      (2) Right and left renal artery
      (3) Right and left iliac artery
      (4) Right and left femoral artery
   b) Note normal findings: no bruits, although systolic bruits may be heard over aorta and over iliac and femoral arteries.
   c) Document abnormal findings: bruits with systolic and diastolic components.
      (1) Over arteries, bruits may indicate aneurysm or stenosis.
      (2) A hepatic bruit may indicate alcoholic hepatitis or a liver tumor.

3. Friction rubs (scratchy, scraping sounds that vary with respiration)
   a) Auscultate with diaphragm of stethoscope over liver or spleen.
   b) Note normal findings: no rubs.
   c) Document abnormal findings: Rubs may indicate liver tumor, peritonitis, gonococcal hepatitis, or splenic infarction.

4. Venous hum (continuous soft humming sound)
   a) Auscultate with bell and diaphragm over epigastric and umbilical regions.
   b) Note normal findings: Hum may be heard over inferior vena cava.
   c) Document abnormal findings: Hum over liver or spleen may indicate hepatic cirrhosis or angiomas.

D. Percussion (see section III,D,2 of Chapter 6 for techniques)
   1. Percuss all 4 quadrants lightly and systematically to note alternation of tympany and dullness; tympany usually heard over most of abdomen; solid masses percuss with a dull sound.
   2. Assess liver size.
      a) Lower border
         (1) Begin along right midclavicular line below umbilicus in area of tympany; percuss upward until dull note is heard.
         (2) Mark as lower border of liver.
         (3) Scratch test can also be used to assess lower border.
            (a) Place diaphragm of stethoscope at midclavicular line just above right costal margin.
            (b) With fingernail, lightly scratch skin along midclavicular line from below umbilicus to costal margin.
            (c) When finger reaches edge of liver, examiner will hear scratching through stethoscope.

b) Upper border
    (1) Begin in area of lung resonance along right midclavicular line and percuss downward until dull sound is heard.
    (2) Mark as upper border.
c) Measure distance (in cm) between marks: Normal vertical span at right midclavicular line is 6–12 cm.

3. Assess spleen size.
  a) Dullness of normal spleen may be difficult to locate between lung resonance and abdominal tympany; may be found in area of ninth to 11th rib just posterior to midaxillary line.
  b) To assess possibility of splenomegaly, percuss the lowest left intercostal space at anterior axillary line; ask client to take and hold a deep breath as you percuss; dull note on inspiration indicates splenic enlargement.

4. Percuss for ascites.
  a) Shifting dullness
    (1) With client supine, percuss from umbilicus outward; mark points where tympany changes to dullness.
    (2) Have client turn on side facing examiner; repeat percussion and mark borders; relatively constant borders indicate lack of ascites, borders that shift to dependent side indicate presence of ascites.
  b) Fluid wave
    (1) Have client or assistant press ulnar edge of hand firmly into middle of client's abdomen.
    (2) Tap opposite flank sharply with fingertips; if ascites are present, impulse will be transmitted through fluid to hand pressed on opposite side of abdomen.

D. Palpation
  1. Techniques (client supine)
    a) Light palpation
      (1) Technique is used to identify muscular resistance, areas of tenderness, and superficial organs and masses.
      (2) With forearm horizontal, hand flat on abdomen, and fingers together, gently palpate all 4 quadrants with a light, dipping motion, depressing abdomen up to 1 cm (examine areas of tenderness last).
      (3) If resistance occurs, ask client to exhale deeply through the mouth to relax rectus muscles, then palpate again; continuing resistance may indicate peritonitis.
    b) Deep palpation
      (1) Technique is used to detect and explore abdominal masses and organs that lie deeper in abdomen.
      (2) Apply pressure through fingers up to depth of 4 cm (more for obese client).
      (3) Palpate all 4 quadrants; note location, size, shape, consistency, tenderness, and mobility of masses and organs.

              (4) Where necessary, use bimanual palpation (1 hand on top of the other); upper hand applies pressure and lower hand feels abdomen.

              (5) When client reports pain, test for rebound tenderness: Slowly but firmly press fingers deep into abdomen and quickly release pressure; increased pain with release indicates peritoneal inflammation.

       c) Ballottement

              (1) Technique is used to assess floating object.

              (2) Straighten fingers of hand, place on abdominal surface, and make swift bouncing movement over organ or mass; technique will briefly displace fluid to allow fingers to feel surface of structure through abdominal wall.

    2. Palpating abdominal organs

       a) The liver (client supine)

              (1) Place left hand on client's back beneath the right 11th and 12th ribs so that client relaxes against palm of hand; place right hand parallel to right costal margin in the midclavicular line.

              (2) Ask client to breathe deeply; pressing gently inward and up, feel liver as it descends on inspiration, releasing pressure slightly so that organ can slip under fingertips; palpate anterior surface and assess size and firmness.

              (3) May use hooking technique: Place both hands side by side below area of liver dullness and instruct client to breathe deeply; press fingers in and upward, attempting to feel liver with fingertips of both hands.

              (4) Use fist (blunt) percussion to assess tenderness.

                 (a) Place 1 hand flat over region of liver dullness.

                 (b) Strike back of flat hand with the fist of other hand.

                 (c) Pain or muscle guarding may indicate hepatitis or cholecystitis.

       b) The spleen: 2 positions

              (1) Client supine, examiner at client's right

                 (a) Reach with left hand over abdomen to client's back; press lower left rib cage forward (displaces spleen anteriorly).

                 (b) Place right hand flat on abdomen in left upper quadrant (LUQ); push fingers beneath costal margin toward spleen.

                 (c) Ask client to breathe deeply; try to feel tip of spleen as it moves toward fingers (spleen normally not palpable).

                 (d) Note tenderness, contour, and distance beneath left costal margin; more than 1 cm indicates splenomegaly.

   (2) Client on right side, hips and knees flexed slightly: Repeat procedure above.
  c) The kidneys: client supine, examiner on client's right
   (1) Palpate left kidney (not normally palpable).
    (a) Reach across client with left arm, elevate left flank (displaces kidney anteriorly).
    (b) Place right hand on abdomen; use deep palpation in LUQ as client inhales deeply.
   (2) Palpate right kidney: Repeat previous procedure but on right side; kidney not usually palpable but may feel lower pole of right kidney as smooth, round mass in thin adults or elderly clients.
   (3) Note size and contour of kidney if palpable.
 3. Palpating to assess for specific conditions
  a) Acute cholecystitis: Assess for Murphy's sign.
   (1) Hook thumb or fingers deep beneath right costal margin and ask client to inhale deeply.
   (2) Sharply increased tenderness and stopped inspiration are positive Murphy's sign, suggesting acute cholecystitis.
  b) Appendicitis
   (1) Rovsing's sign: Press firmly in left lower quadrant (LLQ) and quickly release pressure; pain referred to right lower quadrant (RLQ) suggests appendicitis.
   (2) Psoas sign: With client's legs extended, place hand just above client's right knee and ask client to raise thigh against hand's pressure; increased abdominal pain in lower quadrants suggests appendicitis.
   (3) Obturator sign: Flex client's right hip and knee to 90°; rotate leg internally; right hypogastric pain suggests appendicitis.

IV. Essential nursing care for client with abdominal pain

See text pages
_____

A. Nursing assessment
 1. Gather relevant health history information (same as section I of this chapter).
 2. Before beginning assessment, ask client to identify areas of pain or tenderness; assess these areas last.
 3. Inspect abdomen for asymmetry, visible peristaltic waves, and masses.
 4. Auscultate bowel sounds.
 5. Palpate lightly with fingertips to delineate the area of tenderness; check for rebound tenderness.

B. Nursing diagnoses
 1. Altered role performance related to abdominal pain
 2. Altered nutrition, less than body requirements, related to abdominal pain
 3. Altered self-care related to knowledge deficit concerning causes of abdominal pain
 4. Anxiety related to uncertainty about cause of abdominal pain as expressed by client

C. Nursing implementation (intervention)
1. Offer information about client's medical diagnosis.
2. Educate client concerning treatment and prognosis.
3. Help client to determine lifestyle modifications that may help avoid recurrence of abdominal pain.

D. Nursing evaluation
1. Client demonstrates through verbalization an understanding of disorder and treatment.
2. Client demonstrates decreased anxiety and an understanding of condition and treatment.
3. Client reports return to normal eating habits and participation in usual activities.

1. During the assessment of the abdomen the nurse should ask the client about her/his use of over-the-counter (OTC) and prescription medications because:

    a. The types of medications may reveal an abdominal disorder the client has not mentioned.

    b. Many medications taken orally will affect gastrointestinal (GI) function.

    c. The nurse may be able to provide education about the medications the client is taking.

    d. The nurse can identify interactions between medications the client is taking.

2. A 56-year-old male client presents with "heartburn." Which of the following questions should the nurse ask next in order to gather additional data about this complaint?

    a. "Does the pain keep you from performing your normal daily activities?"

    b. "Are you having any difficulty with body movement or joint pain?"

    c. "Do any other symptoms accompany this pain?"

    d. "Have you had abdominal surgery?"

3. A 19-year-old male client complains of right lower quadrant abdominal pain. Which of the following is the nurse's priority action?

    a. Auscultate bowel sounds in the right lower quadrant.

    b. Palpate the right lower quadrant firmly to check for rebound tenderness.

    c. Obtain the client's dietary history and calculate fluid and calorie intake for the previous day.

    d. Question the client about what symptoms accompany the pain.

4. The nurse is assessing the abdomen of a 32-year-old obese female client. Upon inspection the nurse notes a bulge radiating upward above the umbilicus. Palpation with the index finger reveals a ring of tissue with a soft center. These findings point most clearly to:

    a. An umbilical hernia.

    b. An epigastric hernia.

    c. Ascites.

    d. A liver tumor.

5. Which of the following should the nurse keep in mind when auscultating the abdomen?

    a. Auscultation provides little useful information in a client who has no GI symptoms.

    b. Auscultation provides information about bowel motility and the underlying vessels and organs.

    c. Vascular sounds such as bruits and friction rubs are normally heard during auscultation of the abdomen.

    d. The absence of bowel sounds during auscultation constitutes an emergency and should be reported to a physician without delay.

6. The nurse is performing an assessment on a 65-year-old male client with an early bowel obstruction. Which of the following findings should the nurse expect to find?

    a. During inspection of the abdomen, visible peristaltic waves are absent.

    b. During auscultation of the abdomen, rushing, high-pitched sounds coincide with an abdominal cramp.

    c. During auscultation of the abdomen, bowel sounds are absent in the lower quadrants.

    d. During palpation of the abdomen, a firm mass may be felt at the site of the obstruction.

7. The nurse is percussing the abdomen of a 62-year-old male client who has been diagnosed with emphysema. The nurse finds

that the upper border of the liver is low and the liver span at the right midclavicular line is 12 cm. The liver is palpable below the costal margin. Her assessment findings indicate:

a. A liver of normal size that has been displaced downward.
b. An enlarged, irregular liver that suggests malignancy.
c. A friction rub caused by gonococcal hepatitis.
d. Hepatomegaly caused by cirrhosis.

8. The nurse has just finished assessing the abdomen of a 72-year-old female client. Which of the following findings should be immediately reported to the physician?

a. Identified on percussion: dullness in the right upper quadrant
b. Identified on percussion: tympany in the left upper quadrant
c. Identified on palpation: a round mass, pulsating slightly, in the mid-epigastric region
d. Identified on palpation: a firm rounded mass midline in the hypogastric region

9. The nurse is having difficulty palpating the spleen while doing an abdominal assessment of a 64-year-old female client. Which of the following actions may assist the nurse in successfully palpating the spleen?

a. Position the client prone and ask the client to breathe deeply and slowly.
b. Position the client supine and ask her to exhale completely and then hold her breath.
c. Assist the client onto her left side with her knees and hips flexed slightly.
d. Assist the client onto her right side with her knees and hips flexed slightly.

10. A 46-year-old male client complains of cramping abdominal pain, nausea, and constipation. Palpation reveals tenderness in the left lower quadrant. These assessment findings point most clearly to:

a. Acute pancreatitis.
b. Acute diverticulitis.

c. Acute appendicitis.
d. Acute cholecystitis.

11. A 45-year-old female client presents with complaints of a steady epigastric pain with nausea, vomiting, and a mild fever. Which of the following statements by the client would point more clearly to pancreatitis than another abdominal disorder?

a. "The pain gets worse when I lie down."
b. "I probably don't eat enough fresh fruit and vegetables."
c. "All day I've had indigestion and I can't stop belching."
d. "I've felt so depressed in the past week or so."

12. You are performing an assessment of a 42-year-old male client who was recently hospitalized with a diagnosis of a peptic ulcer. Which of the following statements by the client indicates the need for further teaching?

a. "I know that cutting down on some of the stress in my life will help me stay out of the hospital."
b. "I'll cut down on my smoking, maybe even stop entirely."
c. "I should consult my doctor before I take any oral medications."
d. "Often I don't have time for breakfast, but I usually manage to have at least a cup of coffee in the morning."

ANSWERS

1. **Correct answer is b.** Medications taken orally can cause adverse reactions such as nausea, vomiting, diarrhea, constipation, and gastritis.

a. Although it is possible that the nurse will gain information about abdominal function from the answer to this question, it would not be the primary reason for asking the question.
c. While the nurse may act in this role, this would not be the primary reason for asking this question.

d. While the nurse may be able to identify possible interactions between drugs, this is not the nurse's primary reason for asking this question.

2. **Correct answer is c.** "Heartburn" is a symptom that can have a number of causes, some more serious than others. The nurse will want to find out what other symptoms accompany this pain to begin to narrow the possibilities.

   a. This question helps to assess the client's ability to maintain activities of daily living (ADLs). It may be a useful question to ask later, but questions that help to clarify the source of the pain are more beneficial at this point.
   b. This question would be helpful if the nurse suspected Crohn's disease. The client's complaint, however, does not lead first to this finding.
   d. This information is useful to the nurse in collecting health history information for an abdominal assessment. It is not, however, directly related to the client's complaint.

3. **Correct answer is d.** Before beginning the physical assessment of this client, the nurse must gather additional data about the complaint. The nurse should begin with symptoms (nausea, vomiting, diarrhea, constipation) that may accompany the pain.

   a. Bowel sounds should be auscultated in all 4 quadrants, but this should be done after gathering data about the complaint.
   b. The abdomen should be palpated gently and after auscultation.
   c. Some of this information may be needed to determine intake and output status but this is not priority information at the beginning of the exam.

4. **Correct answer is a.** These findings are most consistent with an umbilical hernia, in which abdominal tissue protrudes through a defective umbilical ring. In a child umbilical hernias usually protrude at the umbilical opening. In adults the bulge is usually seen above the umbilicus. The umbilical ring can be palpated.

   b. An epigastric hernia is usually seen higher in the abdomen, nearer to the xiphoid process. The umbilical ring would not be palpable with an epigastric hernia.
   c. Ascites is an accumulation of fluid within the abdominal cavity. Distension of the abdomen, not a localized bulge, would appear.
   d. The liver is located higher in the abdomen, not at the level of the umbilicus.

5. **Correct answer is b.** Auscultation is performed to provide information about bowel motility and to assess the client for vascular abnormalities. Bowel sounds can be heard throughout the abdomen, but the nurse should listen in specific areas for vascular sounds.

   a. Even in the absence of specific GI symptoms, the abdomen should always be auscultated.
   c. Bruits are not normally heard during auscultation of the abdomen. Friction rubs are not vascular sounds; they result from 2 inflamed surfaces rubbing together.
   d. The absence of bowel sounds during an exam may be related to a full bladder or may have some other simple explanation. Further data should be gathered about the client before reporting this finding.

6. **Correct answer is b.** An early bowel obstruction often produces high-pitched, tinkling sounds or high-pitched rushing sounds accompanying an abdominal cramp. In a late obstruction, sounds may be absent in all quadrants.

   a. If the client has a bowel obstruction, increased peristaltic waves may be visible above the obstruction.
   c. In an early bowel obstruction, high-pitched sounds are common. In a late bowel obstruction, sounds will be absent in all quadrants.
   d. It is not possible to palpate a bowel obstruction.

7. **Correct answer is a.** The nurse has noted the low upper border of the liver; the low diaphragm present with emphysema will displace the liver downward. The liver, with a span of 12 cm, is of normal size for an adult male.

b. The assessment findings did not indicate liver enlargement or the irregularity associated with malignancy.
c. A friction rub is detected through auscultation, not through percussion or palpation.
d. The liver is not enlarged; a 12 cm span is within the normal range for an adult male.

8. **Correct answer is c.** This mass could be a dissecting aortic aneurysm because of its location and pulsation. Palpating it further could cause a rupture.

a. The nurse has identified the liver.
b. The nurse has identified the air-filled stomach.
d. The nurse has probably identified the uterus or a full bladder.

9. **Correct answer is d.** In this position, gravity may bring the spleen forward and to the right so it can be palpated.

a, b, and **c.** None of these positions will facilitate the palpation of the spleen.

10. **Correct answer is b.** These signs and symptoms all indicate acute diverticulitis. Sometimes vomiting occurs as well. The sigmoid colon is most often affected by diverticulitis.

a. The pain of acute pancreatitis is epigastric or in the left upper quadrant. Nausea and vomiting also occur.

c. Many of these symptoms apply to appendicitis, but the pain of appendicitis is at first generalized and eventually settles in the right lower quadrant.
d. The pain of acute cholecystitis is epigastric or in the right upper quadrant. The enlarged gallbladder is usually palpable and tender.

11. **Correct answer is a.** The pain of acute pancreatitis becomes worse when the client is supine. Leaning forward with the trunk flexed may relieve the pain somewhat.

b. Persons with diets low in fiber are not at a high risk for pancreatitis, although they may be at risk for other disorders such as diverticulitis. Furthermore, the pain of diverticulitis is located in the left lower quadrant.
c. Persons with these symptoms may have a peptic ulcer or dyspepsia. These symptoms are not specific to pancreatitis.
d. Emotional stress is not linked to pancreatitis. It could, however, be a factor in diseases such as ulcerative colitis or Crohn's disease.

12. **Correct answer is d.** High intake of caffeine, especially on an empty stomach, can aggravate a peptic ulcer. The nurse should explain this to the client and suggest alternatives.

a. The client understands the potential link between emotional stress and the aggravation of this condition.
b. The client understands that cigarette smoking may aggravate this condition.
c. The client understands that he should consult his physician before taking oral medications because of the adverse effects they may have on his condition.

10

The Musculoskeletal System

OVERVIEW

I. **Relevant health history**
  A. Current status
  B. Past status
  C. Family history

II. **Anatomy and physiology**
  A. Bones
  B. Joints
  C. Cartilage
  D. Muscles, tendons, and ligaments

III. **Assessment techniques**
  A. Approach
  B. General inspection

  C. Inspection and palpation of bones
  D. Inspection and palpation of joints
  E. Inspection and palpation of muscles

IV. **Essential nursing care for client with joint pain**
  A. Nursing assessment
  B. Nursing diagnoses
  C. Nursing implementation (intervention)
  D. Nursing evaluation

NURSING HIGHLIGHTS

1. During inspection and palpation, proceed from head to toe and compare all bilateral structures to detect asymmetry, atrophy, or hypertrophy.
2. Before palpating, especially the joints, ask the client if there is any pain or tenderness. If so, palpate lightly and gently.

GLOSSARY

crepitation—abnormal grating or crackling sounds produced when bone surfaces rub together; also called crepitus
dorsiflexion—backward bending
external rotation—turning of a limb away from the midline of the body
goniometer—instrument used to measure range-of-motion angles of a joint
internal rotation—turning of a limb toward the midline of the body

ENHANCED OUTLINE

I. Relevant health history

See text pages
_____

A. Current status
  1. Does the client have pain in any joint or muscle?
     a) Location
     b) Description (e.g., stabbing, throbbing, dull, numbing, prickling, cramping, burning)
     c) Onset (approximate date; gradual or sudden)
     d) Palliative or provocative factors
     e) Treatments
  2. Does client have any other joint symptoms (e.g., popping, stiffness, grating, swelling, redness)
  3. Does client have other muscle symptoms (e.g., weakness, swelling)?

B. Past status
  1. Has the client ever had a serious joint, muscle, ligament, or bone injury?
     a) Treatment
     b) Residual effects (e.g., stiffness or restricted motion)
  2. Has the client ever had surgery involving a bone, muscle, or joint?
     a) Purpose of surgery (e.g., relief of pain or correction of deformity)
     b) Residual effects
  3. Has the client had any recent changes in strength or coordination?

C. Family history: Has anyone in the client's family been diagnosed with osteoporosis, arthritis, gout, or muscular dystrophy?

II. Anatomy and physiology

See text pages
_____

A. Bones
  1. Functions
     a) To protect internal organs and tissues
     b) To support and stabilize soft tissue of body
     c) To provide surface for attachment of muscles, ligaments, and tendons
     d) To allow movement using mechanical principles
     e) To produce red blood cells and store energy in marrow
     f) To store minerals such as calcium and phosphorus
  2. Classification
     a) By shape (e.g., long, short, flat, irregular, sesamoid)
     b) By location: 2 main divisions of skeleton
        (1) Axial skeleton: bones near longitudinal axis including skull, vertebrae, ribs, sternum

   (2) Appendicular skeleton: bones farther from axis including bones of extremities
 3. Growth
  a) Growth occurs in circumference and length until about age 18–20.
  b) Throughout life, old bone tissue is replaced and new tissue is formed (remodeling).

B. Joints (articulations)
 1. Functions: to connect bone to bone and facilitate movement
 2. Classification: by extent of movement and mechanical principle
  a) Synarthrodial joints (e.g., cranial sutures)
   (1) Joints are non-moveable.
   (2) Bones are held together by thin layer of fibrous connective tissue.
  b) Amphiarthrodial joints (e.g., symphysis pubis)
   (1) Joints are slightly moveable.
   (2) Bones are held together with cartilage.
  c) Diarthrodial (synovial) joints (e.g., ankle, wrist, knee, hip)
   (1) Joints are freely moveable.
   (2) Cavity between bones forms joint.
    (a) Cavity lined with synovial membrane and hyaline cartilage (at bone ends); secretes lubricating synovial fluid.
    (b) Fibrous joint capsule surrounds cavity; ligaments, tendons, and muscles stabilize joint.
   (3) There are 5 basic types of synovial joints.
    (a) Hinge joints (e.g., elbow, knee, ankle)
    (b) Pivot (e.g., radioulnar)
    (c) Saddle joints (e.g., thumb)
    (d) Gliding joints (e.g., carpal, tarsal)
    (e) Ball-and-socket joints (e.g., shoulder, hip)
 3. Bursae
  a) Fluid-filled synovial sacs located in and around joints to reduce friction and facilitate movement; act as cushions
  b) Most common sites: shoulder, elbow, knee, hip, heel

C. Cartilage: strong, fibrous connective tissue
 1. Functions
  a) To support and shape soft tissue
  b) To cushion and absorb shock
 2. Classification
  a) Fibrous (symphysis pubis, intervertebral disks, knee menisci)
  b) Hyaline (covers articular bone surfaces; connects ribs to sternum; appears in trachea, bronchi, nasal septum)
  c) Elastic (auditory tubes, external ear, epiglottis)

D. Muscles, tendons, and ligaments
 1. Muscle function: to produce motion through contraction
 2. Muscle classification
  a) Visceral muscle (smooth, involuntary): lines walls of blood vessels and most abdominal organs

      b) Skeletal muscle (striated, voluntary): attached to bones; produces motion through contraction

      c) Cardiac muscle (striated, involuntary): found only in heart

   3. Tendons: fibrous bands of connective tissue that attach muscles to bones and allow bones to move when muscles contract

   4. Ligaments: fibrous bands of connective tissue that bind bones to bones at joints and connect cartilage together; provide support and strength to joints and limit motion

III. Assessment techniques

See text pages

A. Approach
   1. Provide warmth and privacy (client may wear underwear or swimwear).
   2. Gather equipment: tape measure and goniometer.
   3. Watch for signs of fatigue, discomfort, or unsteadiness.

B. General inspection: Note movements of client from the time client or examiner enters room.
   1. Posture: Client stands straight and examiner views body alignment from all sides.
      a) Normal findings: Consider racial differences (e.g., pronounced lumbar lordosis in some blacks).
         (1) Convex curvature of thoracic spine and concave curvature of cervical and lumbar spine
         (2) Symmetry of shoulders, scapulae, and iliac crests
      b) Abnormal findings
         (1) Scoliosis: lateral deviation of spine; easily observed from behind while client bends to touch toes
         (2) Kyphosis: abnormal flexion of spine; rounded thoracic spine convexity common in elderly women
         (3) Lordosis (swayback): abnormal extension of spine, usually of lumbar region; common in toddlers and during latter stages of pregnancy
         (4) Asymmetry of shoulders, scapulae, or iliac crests
         (5) Genu valgum (knock knees): lateral deviation of legs toward midline; common in child beginning to walk
         (6) Genu varum (bowlegs): lateral deviation of legs away from midline; common in preschool children
   2. Gait: Barefoot client walks away, turns around, walks back while examiner observes.
      a) Normal findings: stages of normal gait
         (1) Stance phase: brief period while both feet are on ground
            (a) Heel strike: Heel contacts floor or ground; should be quiet and coordinated.

      (b) Midstance: Body weight is transferred from heel to ball of foot; foot should support weight evenly.

      (c) Push off: Heel leaves ground; toes should be flexed and lift should be smooth.

    (2) Swing phase

      (a) Acceleration: Quadriceps muscle contracts to initiate extension of leg and forward swing.

      (b) Midswing (swing through): Lifted foot travels ahead of weight-bearing foot; foot should clear ground.

      (c) Deceleration: Hamstring muscles contract to inhibit forward swing in preparation for heel strike.

    (3) Coordinated, rhythmic, balanced, smooth gait

    (4) Developmental variations: waddling gait of late pregnancy; gait of elderly with short, uncertain steps and some shuffling

  b) Abnormal findings: dragging or slapping of feet, abnormally wide support base, staggering, lurching (see section III,C,2,a of Chapter 12)

C. Inspection and palpation of bones

  1. Inspect bones: Take measurements.

    a) Measure client's height (see section I,E of Chapter 2).

    b) Measure extremities: client supine on flat surface with arms and legs extended.

      (1) Arms: Measure from tip of acromion process to tip of middle finger.

      (2) Legs: Measure from lower edge of anterosuperior iliac spine to tibial malleolus.

    c) Document abnormal findings: more than 1 cm disparity between corresponding limbs.

  2. Palpate to assess presence of tumors, fractures, tenderness, or pain.

D. Inspection and palpation of joints

  1. General technique

    a) First inspect joints for swelling, redness, deformity, subcutaneous nodules, or tumors.

    b) Palpate for pain, tenderness, swelling, increased temperature, crepitation, stiffness, or deformity.

    c) Assess range of motion with goniometer.

  2. Temporomandibular joint

    a) Palpate with fingertips anterior to external meatus of ear while client opens and closes jaw; there should be no tenderness and jaw movement should be smooth and painless.

    b) Assess range of motion: opening and closing of jaw (normal distance between upper and lower incisors is 3–6 cm), protrusion, retrusion, lateral motion.

  3. Cervical spine

    a) Palpate spinous process of cervical spine for tenderness.

    b) Assess range of motion: flexion (45°), extension (50°–55°), lateral rotation (70° left and right), lateral bending (40° left and right).

I. Relevant health history	II. Anatomy and physiology	III. Assessment techniques	IV. Essential nursing care for client with joint pain

4. Shoulder (glenohumeral) joint
   a) Standing face to face with client, palpate for tenderness with thumb on anterior and fingertips on posterior aspect as client adducts arm and then moves humerus backward 20°.
   b) Assess range of motion: forward flexion (180°); backward flexion (50°–60°); rotation, external and internal (90°); abduction (180°); adduction (45°–50°).

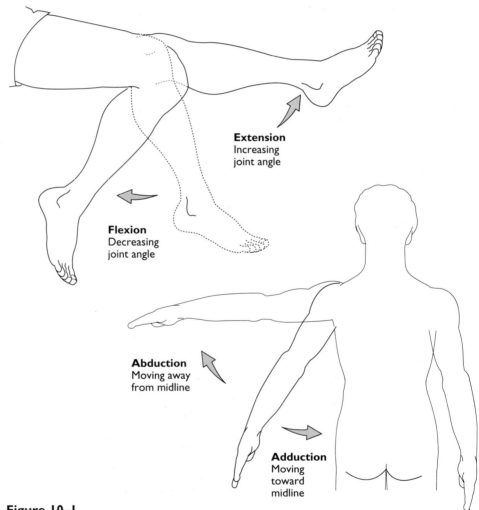

Extension
Increasing joint angle

Flexion
Decreasing joint angle

Abduction
Moving away from midline

Adduction
Moving toward midline

Figure 10–1
Joint Movement

5. Elbow joint
   a) Palpate with fingertips on posterior aspect and thumb applying pressure on anterior aspect while client's arm is flexed 70°; note nodules or swelling.
   b) Assess range of motion: supination (90°), pronation (90°), flexion (150°–160°).
6. Wrist joint
   a) Palpate using both hands with thumbs on dorsum and index fingers beneath wrist; note swelling, tenderness.
   b) Assess range of motion: dorsiflexion (70° above horizontal), flexion (80°–90° below horizontal), lateral (30°–50° ulnar deviation and 20° radial deviation).
7. Carpal, metacarpal, and phalangeal joints
   a) Palpate with thumbs and index fingers for swelling, bony enlargement.
   b) Assess range of motion.
      (1) Metacarpophalangeal (MCP) joint: flexion (90°) and dorsiflexion (30° from the extended position)
      (2) Proximal interphalangeal (PIP) joint: flexion (90° from the extended position)
      (3) Distal interphalangeal (DIP) joint: flexion (80°–90° from the extended position
   c) Perform tests for carpal tunnel syndrome.
      (1) Ask client to maintain palmar flexion for 1 minute; numbness and tingling over median nerve is positive Phalen's sign.
      (2) Tap over median nerve (palmar aspect of wrist) in carpal tunnel; tingling or prickling sensation is positive Tinel's sign.
8. Hip joint
   a) Palpation usually not performed except to identify tenderness.
   b) Assess range of motion: abduction (45°–50°), adduction (20°–30°), internal rotation—knee flexed (40°), external rotation—knee flexed (45°), flexion—knee flexed (120°), flexion—knee extended (90°), hyperextension—knee extended (30°).
9. Knee joint
   a) Palpate knee joint.
      (1) For tenderness, warmth
      (2) For effusion: Press down on area just above patella; a bulge at the sides or below the patella indicates effusion.
      (3) Ballottement for floating patella: Apply downward pressure above patella with 1 hand and push patella back against the femur with the other; click indicates floating patella.
   b) Assess range of motion: flexion (120°–130°).
   c) Perform special tests as needed.
      (1) Apley's sign
         (a) With client prone and knee flexed 90°, push down on foot while rotating knee internally and externally.
         (b) Locking or clicks are positive signs of a foreign body in the joint.

          (2) McMurray's sign
             (a) With client supine and knee completely flexed, hold client's knee in 1 hand and heel in the other.
             (b) Internally rotate tibia on femur, then move through 90° and extend fully; repeat with external rotation.
             (c) Audible clicks or inability to extend leg are positive signs of torn meniscus.
    10. Ankle and foot joints
      a) Palpate ankle and metatarsophalangeal joints with thumb and fingers for tenderness.
      b) Assess range of motion.
         (1) Ankle: dorsiflexion (20°), plantar flexion (45°–50°), eversion (20°), inversion (30°), adduction (10°), abduction (20°)
         (2) Metatarsophalangeal joints: dorsiflexion (40°), flexion (40°)

E. Inspection and palpation of muscles: Examine in symmetric pairs.
  1. Inspection
    a) Measure circumference of thigh, calf, and upper arm; use landmarks to ensure measurement of same location on each side.
    b) Document abnormal findings: more than 1 cm disparity between dominant and non-dominant side.
       (1) Atrophy: muscle wasting
       (2) Hypertrophy: excessive muscle size (without history of weight lifting or other body-building exercise)
  2. Palpation: for tone (tension present in resting muscle)
    a) Palpate muscle while at rest and during passive range of motion.
    b) Note normal findings.
       (1) Relaxed muscle is soft, pliable, without tenderness.
       (2) Contracted muscle is firm.
    c) Document abnormal findings.
       (1) Atony (flaccid muscle)
       (2) Hypotonicity (weak muscle)
       (3) Hypertonicity (spastic muscle)
       (4) Fasciculation (muscle twitching)
  3. Tests of muscle strength (See Nurse Alert, "Disorders or Conditions That May Result in Muscle Weakness.")
    a) Have client perform active range-of-motion tests against resistance.
    b) Document according to rating scale.
       (1) Paralysis (0): no muscular contraction
       (2) Severe weakness (1 or T [trace]): slight palpable contraction
       (3) Moderate weakness (2 or P [poor]): active movement only when not opposed by gravity
       (4) Mild weakness (3 or F [fair]): active movement against gravity

(5) Fair (4 or G [good]): active movement against gravity and slight resistance

(6) Normal (5 or N [normal]): active movement against full resistance

IV. Essential nursing care for client with joint pain

A. Nursing assessment
   1. Gather relevant health history information (same as section I of this chapter).
   2. Inspect and palpate joints gently for abnormalities such as warmth, swelling, tenderness, deformity, and nodules.
   3. Assess range of motion for affected joints.

B. Nursing diagnoses
   1. High risk for activity intolerance related to fatigue and pain caused by arthritis
   2. High risk for disuse syndrome related to fatigue and fear of pain caused by arthritis
   3. Self-care deficit in dressing and grooming related to difficulty in using hands because of arthritis
   4. Altered activities of daily living (ADLs) related to chronic pain

C. Nursing implementation (intervention)
   1. Provide information to client regarding medical diagnosis, treatment, and prognosis.
   2. Teach client range-of-motion exercises for the affected joints.
   3. If appropriate, discuss a weight control program to reduce stress on joints.
   4. Refer client to physical therapist for long-term rehabilitation.

D. Nursing evaluation
   1. Client achieves pain relief with prescribed treatment.
   2. Relief of pain allows greater use of limbs and resumption of normal ADLs.
   3. Client performs range-of-motion exercises daily as suggested.

See text pages
_____

1. A 33-year-old male client states during the health history: "I have a lot of pain in my right hip, particularly after I ski." Which of the following questions would be the best one for the nurse to ask next?

   a. "Does anyone in your family have a history of arthritis or other bone, muscle, or joint disease?"
   b. "Do you take the time to warm up and stretch before you begin to ski?"
   c. "Do you have any swelling or weakness along with the pain?"
   d. "Have you ever injured your hip before?"

2. The nurse has just finished an assessment of a 12-year-old female who has a medical diagnosis of scoliosis. Which of the following statements would best explain this diagnosis to the client?

   a. "Scoliosis is an abnormal flexion of your spine. This is why it is difficult for you to stand up straight."
   b. "Scoliosis means that your lower spine curves too far inward. This is why your chest cavity protrudes forward."
   c. "Scoliosis is a lateral deviation of your spine. This is why your hips appear to be misaligned."
   d. "Scoliosis means that your spine curves to one side. This is why your shoulders look uneven."

3. An 8-year-old female client presents to the emergency room with a complaint of pain in her forearm after falling from her bike. Upon inspection of the injury site, the nurse finds no swelling, discoloration, or deformity. Which of the following actions should the nurse take next?

   a. Measure the length of both arms in centimeters and compare the 2 findings.
   b. Assess for point tenderness as well as color, motion, and sensation (CMS) below the site of the injury.
   c. Move the extremity through range-of-motion exercises to assess for crepitus.

   d. Immobilize the injury and prepare the child for an x-ray of the forearm.

4. A 65-year-old female client comes into the clinic complaining of evening joint pain. She has nodules on the dorsolateral aspects of her distal interphalangeal joints. Both middle fingers show a radial deviation of the distal phalanx. These findings best support a diagnosis of:

   a. Rheumatoid arthritis.
   b. Osteoarthritis.
   c. Carpal tunnel syndrome.
   d. Dupuytren's contracture.

5. The nurse is assessing a 52-year-old client who is experiencing shoulder pain. The client's ability to abduct the glenohumeral joint is severely impaired. Which of the following conditions do these findings most clearly indicate?

   a. Kyphosis
   b. Epicondylitis
   c. Rotator cuff tendinitis
   d. Rotator cuff tear

6. The nurse has just completed a full musculoskeletal assessment of a client. Which of the following findings should the nurse report to the physician?

   a. A maximum hip abduction of 35°
   b. A maximum knee flexion of 125°
   c. A maximum ankle dorsiflexion of 20°
   d. A maximum metatarsophalangeal flexion of 40°

7. An 18-year-old male client complains that during a basketball game he had sudden pain in his right knee. He cannot extend the joint fully and the knee "locks" sometimes. Which of the following conditions do these symptoms most clearly point to?

   a. Patellar dislocation
   b. Mild knee sprain
   c. Osteoarthritis
   d. Torn meniscus

8. A 37-year-old female client presents to the clinic with the following signs and symptoms: fever of 102° F and ankle pain. Upon examination the nurse finds that the client's ankle is red, warm, swollen, and extremely tender. Which of the following conditions should the nurse suspect?

   a. Osteomyelitis
   b. Ankylosing spondylitis
   c. Rheumatoid arthritis
   d. Acute gouty arthritis

9. The nurse is performing an assessment of a 17-year-old female client who has been immobilized in a single hip spica cast. In gathering data about the client, which of the following would the nurse want to assess first?

   a. CMS in the casted leg and ROM in the non-casted toes.
   b. The ROM and CMS in the client's upper extremities.
   c. The client's ability to move in bed.
   d. The client's ability to complete self-care.

10. The nurse is performing an assessment on a 30-year-old female client who has recently been treated for low back pain that occurred as a result of an automobile accident. Which of these statements indicates the client's need for further education?

    a. "If I have pain that radiates down my leg, I should come back in to the clinic."
    b. "If I need it, I can take this over-the-counter pain medication every 4 hours."
    c. "As long as I have no back pain, I can lift my daughter."
    d. "I need to watch my diet so I don't gain weight while I am off work."

11. A 20-year-old male client presents with complaints of generalized muscle weakness in his legs. Which of the following actions should the nurse perform first?

    a. Observe the client for hypertonicity and fasciculation.
    b. Palpate the muscle while the client is at rest.
    c. Measure the client's thighs and calves, comparing the findings.

d. Assess the client's active ROM against resistance.

12. Several months ago the nurse completed an assessment of a 15-year-old female client with a medical diagnosis of muscular dystrophy. The nurse identified "altered activities of daily living (ADLs) related to impaired physical mobility" as the client's primary nursing diagnosis with a goal of returning the client to active participation in ADLs. Which of the following observations from the client's record would provide the most information about the client's progress toward this goal?

    a. Client achieved pain relief with prescribed analgesia.
    b. Client demonstrated use of adaptive devices.
    c. Client performed ROM activities with an increase in repetitions.
    d. Client is able to transfer self with the assistance of 1 person.

ANSWERS

1. **Correct answer is c.** The nurse should follow this statement with a question that allows her/him to obtain more information about the pain itself. This is the answer that most specifically addresses the pain.

   a. Although the nurse will want to ask about the client's family history, this is not the best question for investigating the client's complaint.
   b. Although this question may be important when discussing health promotion activities with the client, this is not the best question for investigating the client's complaint.
   d. Although the nurse will want to know this information, this is not the best question for investigating the client's complaint.

2. **Correct answer is d.** This is an accurate description of the alteration in the spine associated with scoliosis and is presented to

the client in a developmentally appropriate manner.

a. This is a description of kyphosis; also the terminology is at too high a level for this client.
b. This is a description of lordosis.
c. This is an accurate description of the condition, but the terminology is at too high a level for this client.

3. **Correct answer is b.** Many children do not show the same signs of bone trauma as adults do. Because the nurse should suspect a fracture, given the mechanism of injury, she/he would want to assess the integrity of the CMS below the injury site. In addition, many clients with fracture injuries are able to point to the exact place that it hurts.

a. Limb shortening may occur with a displaced fracture. Because there is no deformity noted in the nurse's original assessment, there would be no point in collecting these data.
c. Crepitus is a sign of a fracture; the nurse, however, should not move the injured limb unnecessarily merely to elicit this finding.
d. While these actions will ultimately need to be taken, the nurse should first gather some additional data.

4. **Correct answer is b.** Osteoarthritis, most common among middle-aged and elderly people, presents with hard dorsolateral nodules called Heberden's nodes. The deviation of the distal phalanx to the radial side is also typical, as is pain at night or after exertion.

a. Rheumatoid arthritis commonly involves the proximal or metacarpophalangeal joints rather than the distal interphalangeal joints. The acute form of the disease presents with tender, painful, and stiff joints, often upon waking in the morning.
c. Carpal tunnel syndrome is caused by compression of the median nerve. Although carpal tunnel symptoms are often worse at night, the condition does not produce joint nodules or deviation. Carpal tunnel syndrome symptoms include weakness and pain, numbness, or tingling in the hand.

d. Dupuytren's contracture is a progressive thickening and tightening of the subcutaneous tissue of the palmar surface of the hand. It most often affects middle-aged and older men and if untreated results in flexion of the fourth or fifth fingers. The first symptoms are a thickened plaque overlying the tendon of the ring finger at the distal palmar crease.

5. **Correct answer is d.** Rotator cuff tears occur most often in clients over 40 years old. When there is a rupture at the place where the rotator cuff enters the bone, the arm cannot be abducted. Often the client seems to shrug the shoulder instead of abducting it.

a. Kyphosis is a condition characterized by increased convexity of the thoracic spine. It sometimes produces back pain, but the pain is not concentrated on the shoulder. Also, kyphosis does not create range-of-motion (ROM) problems with the glenohumeral joint.
b. Epicondylitis is characterized by pain and tenderness in the elbow. This condition is caused by repeated strain of the forearm and wrist.
c. Rotator cuff tendinitis usually occurs in younger clients. The arm can usually be abducted, although pain may occur on abduction. This condition can lead to a rotator cuff tear.

6. **Correct answer is a.** The normal ROM for abduction of the hip joint is 45°–50°. Limitation in a client's range of joint motion could indicate a joint disease.

b. This finding is within the normal range (120°–130°) for flexion of the knee joint.
c. This finding is normal for the dorsiflexion of an ankle.
d. This finding is normal for the flexion of metatarsophalangeal joints.

7. **Correct answer is d.** A torn meniscus may occur when the femur is rotated vigorously on the tibia, as might happen when turning in a basketball game. All these manifestations are typical of a torn meniscus. The nurse should use McMurray's sign to assess this condition.

a. A client with patellar dislocation feels the patella dislocate but return to its place when the knee is extended. This client cannot extend the knee.

b. A mild sprain would present pain and swelling but no locking of the joint.

c. Osteoarthritis causes joint pain and limitation of motion, but it is not common among young adults. Also, osteoarthritis does not immediately follow a traumatic injury.

8. **Correct answer is a.** These signs and symptoms are classic indicators of osteomyelitis.

b. Joint swelling and redness are seen in ankylosing spondylitis, and there may be a low fever. The pain is in the spine, however, usually in the lower back or neck. Males between the ages of 10 and 30 are most likely to present symptoms.

c. Although swelling and pain are typical of rheumatoid arthritis, the joint is usually not reddened. Fever may occur, but is not usually this high. Rarely are the ankles the first joints to be affected.

d. Acute gouty arthritis usually presents first in the metatarsophalangeal joints or the dorsum of the foot with swelling, tenderness, redness, and warmth. The presence of tophi confirm this diagnosis. It is a condition most common among middle-aged and older men as well as postmenopausal women.

9. **Correct answer is a.** Before planning care for this client it is important that the nurse obtain baseline information about the client's cast and any effects it is having on her general well-being.

b. While it is important not to overlook other needs the client may have, the upper extremities should not be the primary focus of the nurse's assessment.

c. Application of a hip spica cast leaves the client with little ability to move herself in most ways. While the client's actual abilities need to be assessed, this should not be the focus of the nurse's initial assessment.

d. Application of a hip spica cast leaves the client with limited abilities to meet her self-care needs. While the client's actual abilities need to be assessed, this should not be the focus of the nurse's initial assessment.

10. **Correct answer is c.** The absence of pain does not indicate a problem has resolved. This client needs guidelines for safe lifting.

a. This response indicates the client understands the need to monitor for compression of lumbar nerves, which may indicate a herniated disk.

b. This response indicates the client understands the role of analgesia in her recovery period.

d. This response indicates the client understands the role of excessive weight in the exacerbation of low back pain.

11. **Correct answer is d.** Assessing the client's active ROM against resistance will provide the nurse with information related to the client's current complaint.

a. These observations would provide the nurse with information about the integrity of the muscle while it is at rest. This information would not directly contribute to the database about the client's current complaint.

b. This would provide information about pain. It would be more useful if the client were complaining about muscle pain or cramping.

c. This would provide information about muscle atrophy or hypertrophy. The nurse may want to include this later in the assessment.

12. **Correct answer is c.** The client was able to complete additional repetitions in the ROM activities, indicating an increase in her physical mobility. These changes will allow more active participation in ADLs.

a. This information about the client does not relate to physical abilities.

b and d. This may be an increase in the client's physical mobility but there isn't enough information presented to make this decision.

11

The Reproductive System

OVERVIEW

I. The male reproductive system
  A. Relevant health history
  B. Anatomy and physiology
  C. Assessment techniques

II. The female reproductive system
  A. Relevant health history
  B. Anatomy and physiology
  C. Assessment techniques

III. Essential nursing care for client with suspected benign prostatic hypertrophy
  A. Nursing assessment
  B. Nursing diagnoses
  C. Nursing implementation (intervention)
  D. Nursing evaluation

NURSING HIGHLIGHTS

1. Some clients may refuse to be examined by a practitioner of the opposite sex. (This preference may have a cultural basis.) If this occurs, the nurse should respect the client's wishes and arrange for a different practitioner to do the assessment.
2. Occasionally a male client will have an erection during examination by either a male or a female. The most appropriate response is to reassure him that this is not unusual and to proceed with the examination.
3. Questions about sexual activity should not be asked while the client's genitals are being examined.
4. Some women who have been taught not to touch their genitals may not understand their own anatomy and may be relatively unaware of changes and hesitant to acknowledge them.
5. Tense clients can be taught relaxation techniques to use before and during the examination.

GLOSSARY

anteversion—the normal position of the uterus, in which the body is flexed forward at an acute angle
induration—hardening of tissue, especially skin

retroflexion—acute backward tilt of the body of the uterus toward the rectum
retroversion—tilting backward of the body of the uterus, but at a less acute angle than in retroflexion

ENHANCED OUTLINE

I. The male reproductive system

See text pages

A. Relevant health history
   1. Current status
      a) Does the client have a discharge from the penis?
         (1) Description (e.g., color, consistency, amount, odor)
         (2) Associated symptoms (e.g., pain, burning, itching)
      b) Is the client experiencing any problems with urination (e.g., frequency, difficulty starting stream, changes in amount or color of urine, odor, pain on urination)?
      c) Does the client notice lumps, swelling, lesions, rashes, or areas of tenderness anywhere in the groin?
      d) Is the client experiencing sexual difficulties (e.g., pain, problems with getting or maintaining an erection, premature or delayed ejaculation)?
      e) Is the client taking any medications or undergoing any treatments?
      f) Does the client perform regular testicular self-exams? (See Client Teaching Checklist, "Performing a Testicular Self-Examination.")

✔ CLIENT TEACHING CHECKLIST ✔

Performing a Testicular Self-Examination

Explain to the client how to conduct a testicular self-examination:

1. Perform the self-exam once a month, after a warm bath or shower, when the scrotum is relaxed.
2. Begin by lifting the penis and examining the scrotum for any changes in shape, size, or coloring; the left testicle commonly hangs lower than the right, but note any other signs of asymmetry.
3. Hold the scrotum in the palms of the hands. Examine using the thumbs on top of the scrotum and the fingers underneath. Roll the contents of the scrotum between the thumb and fingers.
4. Roll each testis gently between thumb and fingers, feeling its whole surface; it should be smooth, egg-shaped, rubbery, and easy to move.
5. Identify the epididymis, the crescent on the back of each testis. It should feel soft and spongy and may be tender.
6. Feel the spermatic cord rising up from the epididymis and check for lumps and masses along its length.
7. Report any lumps or masses promptly.

---

2. Past status
   a) Has the client ever had a sore or rash on the penis?
      (1) Description
      (2) Associated symptoms (e.g., pain, discharge)
   b) Has the client ever had a scrotal mass or swelling?
      (1) Description (e.g., size, character, mobility, identification of accompanying pain or tenderness)
      (2) Onset, duration, changes over time
   c) Has the client or his sexual partner ever had a sexually transmitted disease (STD)?
      (1) Identification of disease and any complications
      (2) Treatment
   d) Has the client ever had genitourinary or hernia surgery?
      (1) Type and date of surgery, reason for surgery
      (2) Residual effects
   e) Has the client been diagnosed with cardiovascular disease, neurologic disease, or an endocrine disorder (e.g., diabetes mellitus)?
3. Family history: Has any male in the client's family been diagnosed with prostate cancer, infertility, or a hernia?
4. Developmental considerations: stages of sexual development
   a) Stage 1 (preadolescent): no pubic hair except fine body hair; sexual organs unchanged from childhood proportions
   b) Stage 2
      (1) Pubic hair: sparse growth of lightly pigmented, slightly curling hair at base of penis
      (2) Penis: no enlargement or slight enlargement
      (3) Testes and scrotum: slightly enlarged and reddened with changed texture
   c) Stage 3
      (1) Pubic hair: darker, coarser, curlier; extending over symphysis pubis
      (2) Penis: elongation
      (3) Testes and scrotum: enlargement
   d) Stage 4
      (1) Pubic hair: adultlike coarse and curly hair but not as abundant; not yet present on thighs
      (2) Penis: enlargement, development of glans
      (3) Testes and scrotum: enlarged with darkening of skin
   e) Stage 5: amount and distribution of pubic hair and sexual organs adultlike in appearance

B. Anatomy and physiology
1. Penis: external copulatory organ; allows for urination and ejaculation
   a) Shaft consists of 3 columns of erectile tissue bound together by fibrous tissue.
      (1) 2 corpora cavernosa
      (2) Corpus spongiosum: encases urethra and terminates in cone-shaped extension (glans penis)
   b) Uncircumcised males have a prepuce, or foreskin, partially covering the glans.
2. Scrotum (scrotal sac): supports testes
   a) Pouch consists of outer layer of rough, wrinkled skin over inner muscular layer.
   b) Pouch is divided into 2 parts by septum, each containing a testis (testicle), epididymis, and section of spermatic cord.
3. Testes (testicles): paired ovoid structures (4–5 cm long) suspended in scrotum; produce sperm and secrete testosterone
4. Epididymis: comma-shaped coiled tube on posterolateral and upper surface of each testis that stores, transports, and allows maturation of sperm
5. Vas deferens (ductus deferens): stores and transports sperm from epididymides through ejaculatory duct to urethra
   a) Vas deferens passes from epididymides through inguinal canal to posterior surface of bladder.
   b) Vas deferens together with associated blood and lymphatic vessels, nerves, and muscle comprises spermatic cord.

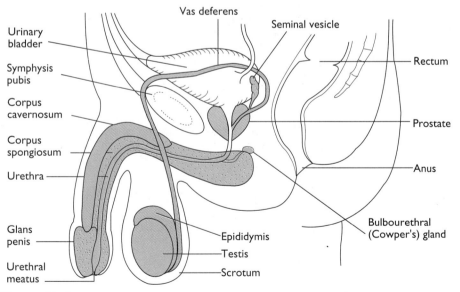

Figure 11–1
Male Reproductive System

      6. Seminal vesicles: pouchlike glands that produce secretions which nourish sperm and become part of semen

      7. Prostate: gland located under bladder and surrounding urethra that produces secretions which become part of semen

  C. Assessment techniques

    1. Approach

      a) Provide privacy; explain all procedures.

      b) Have client urinate before assessment.

      c) Client may be standing or supine for much of assessment.

      d) Always wear gloves.

    2. Inspection and palpation of the penis

      a) Inspect skin of penis, especially glans.

      b) If prepuce is present, ask client to retract it.

        (1) White secretion (smegma) may be evident underneath.

        (2) Return prepuce to usual position before proceeding.

      c) Inspect base of penis and pubic hair for signs of nits or lice.

      d) Note location and form of the urethral meatus.

        (1) Compress glans gently to open urethral meatus and inspect for discharge.

        (2) If client reports discharge and none is observed, have client strip (milk) shaft of penis from base to glans.

        (3) Obtain smear and culture of any discharge.

      e) Palpate shaft with thumb and first 2 fingers; note induration or tenderness.

      f) Document abnormal findings.

        (1) Lesions, ulcers, venereal warts; induration along shaft

        (2) Chancres and signs of carcinoma (sometimes evident under intact prepuce)

        (3) Phimosis: tight prepuce that cannot be retracted

        (4) Paraphimosis: prepuce that will not return to normal position after retraction

        (5) Congenital abnormalities of urethral meatus

          (a) Hypospadias: urethral meatus located on ventral surface of penis

          (b) Epispadias: urethral meatus located on dorsal surface of penis

        (6) Discharge from the penis

    3. Inspection and palpation of the scrotum

      a) Inspect amount and distribution of pubic hair and contours of scrotum (normally asymmetric with left testis lower than right); inspect skin for lesions, swelling.

b) Separate testes with index and middle fingers of 1 hand; palpate scrotum between thumb and fingers of other hand.
    (1) Assess each testis for size, shape, consistency, tenderness, nodules.
    (2) Assess epididymides for size, shape, consistency, tenderness.
    (3) Assess spermatic cords and vas deferentia: Palpate from epididymis to superficial inguinal ring for nodules or swelling.
c) Transilluminate any scrotal swelling: Darken room and shine beam of flashlight from behind scrotum.
    (1) Serous fluid: red glow
    (2) Tissue or blood: no transillumination
d) Document abnormal findings.
    (1) Lesions, induration, inflammation
    (2) Hydrocele
        (a) Hydrocele is accumulation of fluid in tunica vaginalis.
        (b) Examiner can get fingers above mass in scrotum; hydrocele will transilluminate.
    (3) Scrotal hernia
        (a) Scrotal hernia is indirect inguinal hernia.
        (b) Examiner's fingers cannot get above mass in scrotum; scrotal hernia will not transilluminate.
    (4) Varicocele
        (a) Varicose veins of spermatic cord
        (b) Soft, irregular mass; like "bag of worms"
    (5) Tumor
    (6) Sebaceous cysts: firm, yellowish, nontender, cutaneous
    (7) Cryptorchidism: undescended testis

4. Inspection and palpation of the inguinal area for hernias
a) Inspect inguinal and femoral areas for bulges.
    (1) Client should be standing, if able.
    (2) Inspect areas as client holds breath and bears down.
b) Inspect inguinal canal (use right hand for right side, left hand for left side).
    (1) Insert index finger into loose scrotal skin as client flexes ipsalateral knee.
    (2) Follow spermatic cord as far as possible upward to (or through) external inguinal ring (triangular slit).
    (3) Ask client to bear down or cough.
    (4) Soft mass or bulge may indicate hernia.
c) Palpate femoral canal on anterior thigh.
    (1) Canal is located below inguinal ligament and lateral to pubic tubercule.
    (2) Palpate while client strains or bears down; soft mass indicates hernia.

5. Inspection and palpation of the rectum and prostate gland
a) Have client stand with hips flexed, upper body and elbows resting on table; Sims's position may be better for elderly client.

b) Inspect pilonidal area for edema, induration, dimpling, or tenderness.

c) Spread buttocks to expose anus and surrounding area; inspect for fissures, inflammation, lesions, rectal prolapse, hemorrhoids, skin tags, and scars.

d) Insert gloved, lubricated index finger gently into rectum, palmar surface down; palpate all aspects of rectal wall.
   (1) Note nodules, tenderness, irregularities, induration.
   (2) To bring lesion into reach, ask client to bear down; palpate again.

e) Palpate prostate through anterior wall of rectum (the urge to urinate during the examination is normal).
   (1) Normal prostate is smooth, rubbery, nontender, about 2.5–3 cm long and 4 cm in diameter.
   (2) Assess for size, shape, consistency, nodules, tenderness.
   (3) Asking client to bear down allows examiner to palpate masses not otherwise evident.

f) Withdraw finger and inspect feces: Test for occult blood.

g) Document abnormal findings.
   (1) Rectum: nodules, lesions, tenderness, irregularities, induration
   (2) Prostate: tenderness, softness, asymmetry, induration, nodules, protrusion into rectum (enlargement)
       (a) Grade I: <1 cm into rectal lumen
       (b) Grade II: 1–2 cm into rectal lumen
       (c) Grade III: 2–3 cm into rectal lumen
       (d) Grade IV: >3 cm into rectal lumen
   (3) Stool: presence of blood or pus

See text pages
_____

II. The female reproductive system

A. Relevant health history
   1. Current status
      a) What are the client's menses like?
         (1) Cycle description: regular or irregular, cycle length, amount of menses, first day of last menstrual period
         (2) Associated symptoms (e.g., cramping, distension, irritability, mood swings)
         (3) For menopausal client: age menses stopped and associated symptoms
      b) Does the client have a vaginal discharge?
         (1) Description (e.g., color, amount, odor)
         (2) Associated symptoms (e.g., itching, discomfort)

    c) Does the client have lower abdominal pain?

       (1) Location

       (2) Description (e.g., sharp, aching, burning)

       (3) Associated symptoms (e.g., nausea, constipation)

    d) Is the client using a method of contraception?

       (1) Type

       (2) Length of time used

    e) Is the client experiencing sexual difficulties (e.g., pain, decreased libido, bleeding after intercourse)?

    f) What are the date and results of the client's most recent gynecological examination and Pap smear?

2. Past status

    a) At what age did the client's menses begin?

    b) How many pregnancies and live births has the client experienced?

    c) Has the client ever had a miscarriage? If so, during what stage of pregnancy did it occur?

    d) Has the client or her sexual partner ever had a sexually transmitted disease (STD)?

       (1) Identification of disease and any complications

       (2) Treatment

    e) Has the client ever had reproductive surgery?

       (1) Type and date of surgery; reason for surgery

       (2) Residual effects

    f) Has the client ever been diagnosed with endometriosis or had trouble conceiving?

3. Family history

    a) Has any female in the client's family had obstetric problems?

    b) Has any female in the client's family been diagnosed with endometriosis or cancer of any reproductive organ?

    c) Has any family member been diagnosed with diabetes mellitus?

4. Developmental considerations

    a) Assessment of sexual maturity does not depend on internal exam but on growth of pubic hair and development of breasts (see section I,E of Chapter 8).

    b) Range of average menarche is 9–16 years.

    c) Assess stage of sexual development.

       (1) Stage 1 (preadolescent): no pubic hair except fine body hair

       (2) Stage 2: sparse downy hair growing along labia

       (3) Stage 3: darker, coarser, curlier hair occurring sparsely over symphysis pubis

       (4) Stage 4: adultlike hair thicker on symphysis pubis but not yet on thighs

       (5) Stage 5: pubic hair now adultlike in quality and quantity; further spreading up abdomen may occur in mid-twenties

B. Anatomy and physiology

1. External genitalia (vulva or pudendum)

    a) Mons pubis: pad of adipose tissue overlying and protecting symphysis pubis, covered with hair in sexually mature female

   b) Labia: protection for underlying genital structures
    (1) Labia majora: folds of adipose tissue surrounding vestibule and urethral meatus
    (2) Labia minora: thinner mucosal folds within the labia majora; surround vestibule and anteriorly form prepuce of clitoris
   c) Clitoris: structure at anterior angle of vestibule homologous to male glans penis; made of erectile tissue and sensitive to sexual stimulation
   d) Vestibule: cleft within labia minora containing vaginal and urethral orifices
    (1) Introitus: vaginal opening in posterior vestibule
    (2) Hymen: tissue membrane that usually partly covers introitus in virgins; may be ruptured prior to coitus
    (3) Fourchette: posterior boundary of vestibule
   e) Vestibular glands: provide lubrication during intercourse
    (1) Skene's (paraurethral) glands: mucus-producing glands on either side of urethral orifice
    (2) Bartholin's glands: small mucus-producing glands just within posterolateral vaginal orifice

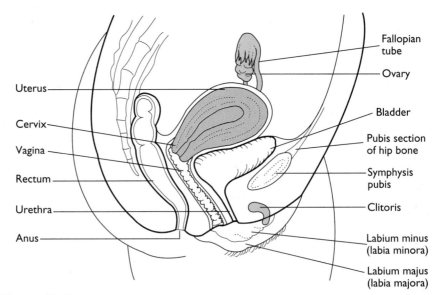

Figure 11–2
Female Reproductive System

  f) Associated structures
   (1) Perineum: area between introitus and anus; term sometimes used to describe entire area from pubic arch to anus
   (2) Urethral orifice or meatus: located within vestibule between clitoris and vagina
 2. Internal genitalia: supported by 4 pairs of ligaments, muscles
  a) Vagina: structure connecting external and internal reproductive organs; passageway for intercourse, menstruation, childbirth
   (1) Elastic muscular tube between urethra and rectum that inclines posteriorly at 45° angle; normally collapsed but capable of distension
   (2) Fornix: recess where cervix protrudes into superior vagina
  b) Uterus: origin of menses; site for development and nourishment of fetus
   (1) Hollow muscular structure shaped like an inverted pear; located between bladder and rectum
   (2) Structure
    (a) Fundus: convex upper surface of corpus that expands to accommodate growing fetus
    (b) Corpus: body of uterus
    (c) Isthmus: narrow region connecting corpus and cervix
    (d) Cervix
     i) Canal-shaped lower end of uterus that opens onto vagina
     ii) Internal cervical os joins isthmus with cervical canal; external cervical os is area where cervix opens into vagina
   (3) Mucosal membrane lining uterus: endometrium
  c) Adnexa
   (1) Fallopian tubes open on fundus of uterus at 1 end and partially surround ovary at the other; fertilization usually occurs in the tube.
   (2) Ovaries are oval organs usually located near lateral pelvic wall; they produce ova and hormones.
C. Assessment techniques
 1. Approach and preparation
  a) Assemble equipment ahead of time: gloves, water-soluble lubricant, several sizes of speculums, Ayre spatula, sterile cotton swabs, glass slides, and cover slides; cytologic fixative, culture bottles or plates; sponge forceps, light source, viewing mirror (for client).
  b) Provide privacy and comfortable room temperature; be sure gloved hands and speculum are warm to the touch.
  c) Have client empty her bladder before examination.
  d) Help client into lithotomy position and drape to cover thighs; elevate head and shoulders to help relax abdominal muscles; arms should be at sides or folded over chest.

e) Explain each step in advance; let client know when you are about to touch her.

2. Inspection and palpation of external genitalia
   a) Assess sexual maturity (see section II,A,4 of this chapter).
   b) Inspect and palpate skin of labia for lesions, excoriations, swelling, and erythema; inspect pubic hairs for nits or lice.
   c) Inspect clitoris, noting size (normally 2 cm or less in length).
   d) Inspect vestibule for erythema and lesions.
   e) Inspect urethral and vaginal orifices and Skene's glands, which should be barely visible unless infected.
   f) Inspect region of Bartholin's glands for inflammation, tenderness, and swelling; if any is evident, palpate area using index finger and thumb.
   g) "Milk" urethra by inserting forefinger into vagina, palmar surface up, and then withdrawing it while pressing gently on anterior surface.
   h) Culture any abnormal discharge found on genitalia or released by milking.

3. Inspection and palpation of internal genitalia
   a) Speculum examination
      (1) Choose size and type of speculum appropriate for client.
      (2) Lubricate speculum only with warm water.
      (3) Place 2 fingers in introitus and press on posterior vaginal wall; with the other hand, gently insert closed speculum downward at a 45° angle to 1 side.
      (4) When blades pass introitus, remove fingers and rotate closed speculum horizontally.
      (5) Open blades and locate cervix, then lock blades open; inspect cervix and cervical mucosa.
      (6) After taking specimens (see section II,C,3,b of this chapter), gently remove speculum, inspecting vaginal walls during removal.
      (7) Recognize normal findings.
         (a) Cervix is pink and free of lesions and growths; color may be purplish in pregnancy.
         (b) Nabothian follicles (small, smooth, round, sometimes yellow) may appear on cervix.
            (i) Caused by cervical gland duct obstruction
            (ii) No pathologic significance in themselves, but sometimes appear with chronic cervicitis
            (iii) Also called Nabothian or retention cysts
         (c) Nulliparous woman has round or oval cervical os; parous woman has irregular or slit-like os.

        (d) Lacerations (stellate or transverse) sometimes appear following difficult deliveries.

        (e) Vaginal walls are pink, transversely rugated; discharge is odorless and non-irritating.

    (8) Document abnormal findings.

        (a) Polyps, lesions, ulcerations, venereal warts

        (b) Purulent discharge

b) Collection of specimens (Pap smear)

    (1) Endocervical smear

        (a) Insert cotton applicator into cervical os.

        (b) Rotate clockwise, then counterclockwise, then remove.

        (c) Paint labeled glass slide with gentle touch to avoid destroying cells and fix.

    (2) Cervical scrape

        (a) Press curved end of Ayre spatula on os of cervix.

        (b) Rotate to scrape cells in a full circle, then remove.

        (c) Apply to labeled glass slide and fix.

    (3) Vaginal smear

        (a) Press cotton applicator at posterior fornix just below cervix (vaginal pool) and roll.

        (b) Apply to labeled glass slide and fix.

c) Bimanual exam

    (1) Insert lubricated finger(s) into vagina with palmar surface toward the anterior vaginal wall; palpate the vaginal wall.

    (2) Gently insert 1 finger tip into external os and move cervix slightly back and forth; assess for contour, consistency, mobility, tenderness, and lesions.

    (3) Place the other hand on abdomen between symphysis pubis and umbilicus; gently apply inward and downward pressure with external hand to allow assessment of uterus.

        (a) Assess position: anteversion, midposition, retroversion, retroflexion.

        (b) Assess for size, contour, consistency, mobility, tenderness, masses.

    (4) Assess right and left adnexa.

        (a) Insert finger into right lateral fornix as external hand on right lower quadrant of abdomen pushes inward and down; repeat on left side.

        (b) Assess for position, size, tenderness, masses.

    (5) Recognize normal findings.

        (a) Cervix: nontender, smooth, and firm (but softened during pregnancy); located along midline of anterior wall or on posterior wall; freely movable 1–2 cm

        (b) Os: firm and open to admit finger approximately 1 cm

        (c) Uterus nontender and freely movable

        (d) Fallopian tubes: not normally palpable

            (e) When palpable, ovaries smooth, firm, ovoid, not larger than 4–6 cm

            (f) Normal vaginal pH: 4.0–5.0

        (6) Document abnormal findings.

            (a) Immobile cervix and uterus; pain with cervical movement

            (b) Myomas (fibroids) or other uterine masses

            (c) Uterine prolapse

            (d) Enlarged fallopian tubes

            (e) Ovarian cysts or tumors

    d) Rectovaginal examination: allows palpation of posterior portion of uterus and rectovaginal septum

        (1) Place a fresh glove on hand used for palpating; lubricate index and middle fingers.

        (2) Ask client to relax her muscles and then bear down.

        (3) Insert index finger into vagina and position it in posterior fornix of cervix as you insert middle finger into rectum.

        (4) Use other hand as in bimanual exam.

        (5) Palpate posterior portion of uterus, rectovaginal septum, and fornix for abnormalities as in bimanual exam.

    e) Anus and rectum: Examine as for male client excluding prostate examination (see section I,C,5 of this chapter).

See text pages
_____

III. Essential nursing care for client with suspected benign prostatic hypertrophy

A. Nursing assessment

    1. Gather relevant health history information (same as section I,A of this chapter).

    2. Perform physical examination, including palpation of prostate (same as section I,C,5 of this chapter).

    3. Evaluate any evident enlargement by estimating number of cm of protrusion into rectum (see section I,C,5,g,2 of this chapter).

B. Nursing diagnoses

    1. Sleep pattern disturbance related to nocturia as revealed by client

    2. Alteration in activities of daily living (ADLs) related to altered urinary elimination (increased frequency) secondary to prostate enlargement

    3. Anxiety related to knowledge deficit concerning condition and prognosis

C. Nursing implementation (intervention)
   1. Explain anatomy of prostate and effects of enlargement on urination.
   2. Explain the treatment options for client's condition.
   3. Instruct client to report any worsening of problem, such as increased frequency and difficulty of urination.

D. Nursing evaluation
   1. Client demonstrates through verbalization an understanding of his condition and prognosis.
   2. Client demonstrates through verbalization an understanding of the rationale for medical treatment and the need to report changes in his condition.

1. The nurse is completing the health history of a 16-year-old male client. In gathering data about the client's reproductive system, which of the following questions would be most important for the nurse to include?

   a. "Do you have any discharge from your penis?"
   b. "Do you perform regular testicular self-examinations?"
   c. "Do you have a family history of prostate cancer?"
   d. "Are you experiencing any sexual difficulties?"

2. The nurse is assessing a 52-year-old male client who is experiencing difficulty with urination. Which of the following questions should the nurse ask to help establish a diagnosis of prostatitis versus benign prostatic hyperplasia?

   a. "Are you experiencing dribbling after you urinate?"
   b. "Are you experiencing any difficulty achieving and maintaining an erection?"
   c. "Are you experiencing fever and/or chills?"
   d. "Have you experienced a change in your libido recently?"

3. A 20-year-old client presents to the college health service with a concern about a sore on his penis. He appears both embarrassed and upset during the interview with the nurse. Which of the following questions or statements provides the best way for the nurse to begin the assessment of this client?

   a. "Did you have unprotected intercourse with someone in the last 6 months?"
   b. "It sounds like you have a sexually transmitted disease. I'll call the doctor in."
   c. "Do you have any pain and burning with urination or discharge from your penis?"
   d. "You sound concerned. Let me ask you some questions about your sexual activity to obtain more information."

4. The nurse is assessing a 46-year-old client who reports that his erections are crooked and often painful. Palpation reveals nontender indurations on the dorsum of the penis. Which of the following conditions should the nurse suspect?

   a. Hypospadias
   b. Genital herpes
   c. Phimosis
   d. Peyronie's disease

5. A 17-year-old client comes into the clinic complaining of acute scrotal pain. Assessment reveals scrotal redness and swelling and testicular retraction. Scrotal elevation does not relieve the pain. What condition do these assessment findings most clearly indicate?

   a. Acute epididymitis
   b. Torsion of the spermatic cord
   c. Varicocele
   d. Testicular cancer

6. The nurse's 39-year-old male client has a medical diagnosis of a direct inguinal hernia. Which of the following should the nurse expect to find on palpation?

   a. A soft mass or bulge palpable above the inguinal ligament near the external inguinal ring
   b. A soft mass or bulge palpable above the inguinal ligament near the internal inguinal ring
   c. A soft mass or bulge palpable in the right lower quadrant of the abdomen
   d. A soft mass or bulge palpable below the inguinal ligament in the femoral canal

7. The mother of a 15-year-old girl has brought her daughter into the clinic. She expresses concern over the fact that her daughter has not begun to have periods. The mother states: "I think there is something wrong with her. My older daughter

started her period at 13." Which of the following should be the priority nursing action?

a. Reassure the mother that there is nothing wrong with her daughter.
b. Obtain a complete and detailed family obstetric history.
c. Assess the adolescent's growth of pubic hair and breast development.
d. Refer the adolescent to an endocrinologist for a further diagnostic workup.

8. A 19-year-old female client presents to the emergency room with a complaint of abdominal pain. Which of the following nursing actions will best help to establish a medical diagnosis of toxic shock syndrome versus pelvic inflammatory disease?

a. Assess the client's temperature and ask her if she has had stomach problems in the past 24 hours.
b. Palpate the abdomen to ascertain degree and location of tenderness.
c. Complete an internal examination noting pain and any vaginal discharge.
d. Complete a health history including first day of last menstrual period (LMP) and type of protection (tampons or absorbent pads) used.

9. Which of the following signs or symptoms is a client diagnosed with endometriosis most likely to report?

a. Pruritus
b. Dysmenorrhea
c. Abdominal pain
d. Fever

10. A 23-year-old client has been diagnosed with vaginal candidiasis. Which of the following assessment findings is most likely in this client?

a. Urinary frequency and urgency
b. Backache in the sacral region
c. Frothy green vaginal discharge
d. White, cheeselike vaginal discharge

11. Palpation of the vagina of a 52-year-old client reveals a bulge in the posterior wall of the vagina. With which of the following conditions is this finding consistent?

a. Cervical eversion
b. Cystocele
c. Rectocele
d. Nabothian follicles

12. A bimanual and rectovaginal examination of a 24-year-old nulliparous female reveals a mobile uterus with a cervix that can be felt through the posterior fornix and a body that can be felt through the rectal wall. The best description for the client's uterine position is:

a. Retroverted.
b. Anteverted.
c. Midposition.
d. Anteflexed.

ANSWERS

1. **Correct answer is a.** An adolescent client will most likely feel quite uncomfortable discussing his genitourinary and sexual functions with the nurse. While it is important for the nurse to complete an examination of the reproductive system, she/he must identify priorities within the information-gathering process. This question will provide crucial information regarding sexually transmitted diseases (STDs). The nurse may need to ask follow-up questions depending upon the client's answer.

b. This question will not yield valuable information. A client of this age may not have been introduced to this procedure. The nurse may want to include this question later to set the stage for health promotion teaching.
c. This is not essential information for a client of this age, who is very unlikely to experience problems with the prostate gland, especially prostate cancer.
d. This is not information the adolescent client will be comfortable discussing with the nurse. It is not appropriate for a client of this age, who may or may not be sexually active.

2. Correct answer is c. Since prostatitis is an infectious process, this is the only question that will differentiate between the 2 diagnoses.

a, b, and **d.** All of these symptoms may be present in either of the 2 conditions.

3. Correct answer is d. This response recognizes the client as an individual. It validates the client's feelings and sets the stage for the remainder of the interview.

a. The nurse will need to know this, but it is a question that should come later in the interview.
b. While this may be the eventual medical diagnosis, it cannot be stated without more data. Stating it at this point will alarm the client unnecessarily.
c. The nurse will need to obtain this information, but this question should be asked later in the process.

4. Correct answer is d. These findings are consistent with Peyronie's disease. Hard, nontender plaques form under the skin on the dorsum of the penis causing bending of the penis during erection and, often, pain upon erection. The client may also report pain during intercourse.

a. Hypospadias is a congenital displacement of the urethral meatus to the ventral surface of the penis. A groove usually is visible running from the opening to the normal location at the end of the penis.
b. Genital herpes presents as a cluster of small vesicles surrounded by erythematous tissue that may erupt into ulcers. The lesions are painful and most often appear on the glans or prepuce. Genital herpes is a viral infection usually transmitted by sexual contact.
c. Phimosis presents as a tight prepuce that cannot be retracted over the glans. Treatment usually consists of circumcision.

5. Correct answer is b. These findings are consistent with torsion, or twisting, of the spermatic cord. This condition occurs most often in adolescents, usually after strenuous exercise or groin trauma. Torsion of the spermatic cord constitutes a surgical emergency.

a. With acute epididymitis the spermatic cord may be thickened and indurated. Scrotal swelling may also occur. The pain is felt primarily along the inguinal canal and may be accompanied by fever. The pain can usually be relieved somewhat with elevation of the scrotum.
c. A varicocele often causes no pain or a dull pain or dragging sensation in the groin. It feels to the examiner like a "bag of worms" that collapses when the scrotum is elevated.
d. A testicular tumor usually presents as a painless mass on the testicle with testicular enlargement.

6. Correct answer is a. A soft mass or bulge at this location most likely indicates a direct inguinal hernia.

b. This finding most clearly indicates an indirect inguinal hernia, which often protrudes into the scrotum. It is most common in infants and in males age 16–20.
c. A mass or bulge in this area may indicate an abdominal hernia, possibly incisional.
d. A mass or bulge in this area may indicate a femoral hernia. This type of hernia is more common among women than among men.

7. Correct answer is c. Assessment of reproductive maturity does not depend on the internal exam but on the growth of pubic hair and development of breasts. Since the normal range for menarche is 9–16 years, absence of menses is not abnormal.

a. Ultimately the nurse may be able to do this, but it is not an appropriate first action. Assessment of sexual maturity is needed. Making this statement at this point would constitute false reassurance of the client and her mother.
b. The nurse will want to obtain this information eventually, but it is not an appropriate first action.
d. The nurse does not have enough data to make a referral at this time.

8. **Correct answer is d.** Toxic shock syndrome has been linked to menstruation and tampon use. Obtaining this information would assist the nurse in differentiating this diagnosis.

   a. The nurse would want to include this but both conditions can produce fever and gastrointestinal (GI) upset.

   b. The nurse may want to include this but both conditions can produce a vague, dull, abdominal pain. In both conditions the client may have trouble localizing the pain.

   c. The nurse may want to include this but the presence or absence of vaginal discharge will not provide the nurse with sufficient data to differentiate between these 2 conditions.

9. **Correct answer is b.** Of the symptoms listed here, dysmenorrhea is the only one specifically associated with endometriosis.

   a. Several conditions, including candidiasis, trichomoniasis, and atrophic vaginitis could present this symptom. It is not, however, associated with endometriosis.

   c. Ovarian cysts, ovarian cancer, and pelvic inflammatory disease may all present with abdominal pain. The pain associated with endometriosis is often referred to the rectum or lower back.

   d. Toxic shock syndrome and pelvic inflammatory disease, among other conditions, may present with a fever. Fever is not, however, associated with endometriosis.

10. **Correct answer is d.** The discharge associated with candidiasis is generally described in this way by clients. It usually has a yeasty odor or may be odorless.

    a. This finding is typical of cystitis or cervicitis.

    b. This finding is typical of endometriosis and sometimes cervicitis.

    c. This finding is typical of trichomoniasis. The discharge is usually malodorous as well.

11. **Correct answer is c.** A rectocele is the protrusion of the rectum into the vagina, caused by weakness of the pelvic muscles. The rectum would protrude through the posterior vaginal wall.

    a. A cervical eversion would be observed during a speculum examination, not during palpation of the vagina. It presents as a velvety red, friable external os.

    b. A cystocele is the protrusion of the bladder into the vagina, caused by weakness of the pelvic muscles. The bulge would appear in the anterior wall of the vagina.

    d. Nabothian follicles (retention cysts) would be observed during a speculum examination, not during palpation of the vagina. They present as small, round, yellowish lesions on the cervix and are caused by cervical gland duct obstruction.

12. **Correct answer is a.** Uterine positions are named for the relationship between the long axis of the uterus and the long axis of the body. A retroverted uterus is tipped backward.

    b. An anteverted uterus is displaced forward. The cervix can be felt through the anterior vaginal wall. Neither the body nor the fundus can be palpated through the rectal wall.

    c. A uterus in midposition has a long axis that is approximately parallel to the long axis of the body. Its cervix can be palpated at the apex of the vagina. The body and fundus may not be palpable at all.

    d. An anteflexed uterus is similar to an anteverted uterus but the fundus is flexed further anteriorly. The cervix can be palpated through the anterior vaginal wall or the vaginal apex; neither the body nor the fundus can be palpated through the rectal wall.

12

The Nervous System

OVERVIEW

I. Relevant health history
  A. Current status
  B. Past status
  C. Family history

II. Anatomy and physiology
  A. Central nervous system (CNS)
  B. Peripheral nervous system

III. Assessment techniques
  A. Approach
  B. Cranial nerve function

  C. Cerebellar function and the motor system
  D. Sensory function
  E. Reflexes

IV. Essential nursing care for client with suspected migraine
  A. Nursing assessment
  B. Nursing diagnoses
  C. Nursing implementation (intervention)
  D. Nursing evaluation

NURSING HIGHLIGHTS

1. The nervous system depends strongly on the proper functioning of certain organs. For example, metabolic imbalances can cause dysfunctions of the nervous system.
2. The extent and focus of the nervous system assessment varies widely depending upon the signs and symptoms reported in the health history.
3. A full neurologic exam may take 2–3 hours and may tire and frustrate the client: Sensitivity and patience are needed.

GLOSSARY

clonus—rapidly alternating involuntary muscular contraction and relaxation
dysarthria—poorly articulated speech

fasciculation—uncontrollable twitching of a muscle group

intention tremor—rhythmic, purposeless movements that are intensified during voluntary movement

stereognosis—ability to recognize objects by touch

ENHANCED OUTLINE

I. Relevant health history

See text pages

A. Current status
1. Does the client have headaches? If so, how would he/she describe them? If they are recurring headaches, at what time of day do they recur? (See Nurse Alert, "Diagnostic Signs of Meningitis.")
2. Does the client ever become dizzy or faint?
3. Does the client have sensory problems?
a) Vision (e.g., blurred or double vision, momentary loss of vision)
b) Hearing (e.g., gradual progressive loss, ringing in ears)
c) Smell (e.g., loss of smell, unusual smells)
d) Taste (e.g., loss of taste, unusual tastes)
e) Touch (e.g., numbness, tingling, decreased sensation)
4. Does the client have any problems with alertness or memory?
5. Does the client have any problems with coordination or balance?
6. Is the client taking any medication to control seizures?

! NURSE *ALERT* **!**

Diagnostic Signs of Meningitis

When a client shows signs of meningitis (e.g., severe headache, vomiting, pain or stiffness in neck), perform the following special assessment techniques:

* Brudzinski's sign: With client supine, place your hands behind the client's head and flex the neck toward the chest; resistance, pain, and the flexing of the hips and knees show positive Brudzinski's sign.

* Kernig's sign: With client supine, flex 1 leg at hip and knee, then straighten knee; resistance and pain show positive Kernig's sign.

B. Past status
1. Has the client ever suffered a head injury?
a) Description and date of injury
b) Treatment and residual effects
2. Has the client ever fainted or blacked out? If so, under what circumstances?
3. Has the client ever had a seizure?
a) Description of seizure and circumstances surrounding it
b) Seizure medication taken
4. Has the client ever had a stroke? If so, when did it occur and what were its effects?

C. Family history: Has a parent or sibling ever had a neurologic disorder (e.g., seizures, brain tumor, degenerative nervous system disease)?

See text pages
_____

II. Anatomy and physiology

A. Central nervous system (CNS): brain and spinal cord
1. Brain
a) Cerebrum: left and right hemispheres, each with 4 major lobes
(1) Frontal lobes: higher thought functions, personality, social behavior
(2) Temporal lobes: hearing, speech comprehension, smell, taste, memory
(3) Parietal lobes: awareness of body position, touch, temperature, pain; interpretation of objects felt with hands
(4) Occipital lobes: interpretation of visual stimuli
b) Cerebellum: coordination, balance, equilibrium
c) Brain stem
(1) Controls respiratory and vasomotor functioning
(2) Origin of most cranial nerves
(3) 3 divisions: midbrain, pons, medulla
d) Diencephalon
(1) Thalamus: relaying of sensory stimuli between spinal cord and cerebrum
(2) Hypothalamus: modulating of temperature, water balance, appetite, pituitary secretions, and autonomic functions
e) Limbic system: associated with emotional responses
2. Spinal cord: part of CNS that controls many reflexes and transmits messages back and forth between brain and peripheral nervous system
a) Slightly flattened cylinder extending from medulla to upper border of second lumbar vertebra; protected by vertebral column

b) Structure: central canal surrounded by H-shaped gray matter, which is surrounded by white matter

B. Peripheral nervous system: sensory and motor nerves and ganglia outside brain and spinal cord
   1. Cranial nerves: 12 pairs of nerves with motor function, sensory function, or both
      a) CN I, olfactory: smell (sensory)
      b) CN II, optic: vision (sensory)
      c) CN III, oculomotor: eye movement (motor)
      d) CN IV, trochlear: eye movement (motor)
      e) CN V, trigeminal
         (1) Stimuli from face, corneal reflex (sensory)
         (2) Mastication (motor)
      f) CN VI, abducens: eye movement (motor)
      g) CN VII, facial nerve
         (1) Taste for anterior two-thirds of tongue (sensory)
         (2) Facial expression, lacrimal glands, closing of eyes (motor)
      h) CN VIII, acoustic (sensory)
         (1) Hearing (cochlear)
         (2) Balance (vestibular)
      i) CN IX, glossopharyngeal
         (1) Taste for posterior one-third of tongue (sensory)
         (2) Swallowing (motor)
      j) CN X, vagus
         (1) Sensations of neck, thoracic, and abdominal regions (sensory)
         (2) Swallowing, gag reflex (motor)
      k) CN XI, spinal accessory: shoulder movement, head rotation (motor)
      l) CN XII, hypoglossal: tongue (motor)
   2. Spinal nerves: transmit impulses to and from body regions
      a) 31 pairs of nerves numbered according to level of cord at which they emerge
         (1) Dorsal: sensory (afferent) neurons that transmit information from receptors to spinal cord and brain
         (2) Ventral: motor (efferent) neurons that transmit information from spinal cord to muscles and parts of body
      b) Reflex arc: simplest route of nerve impulses
         (1) Sensory receptor detects stimulus.
         (2) Sensory neuron carries impulse to spinal cord.
         (3) Sensory neuron synapses with motor neuron.
         (4) Motor neuron transmits impulse to muscle or gland.
         (5) Body part responds.
   3. Autonomic nervous system: regulates involuntary functions
      a) Sympathetic nervous system: excitation
      b) Parasympathetic nervous system: inhibition

See text pages
_____

III. Assessment techniques

A. Approach
  1. Protect client's privacy.
  2. Assess mental status throughout interview and health history (see section III of Chapter 2).
  3. Assemble equipment appropriate for scope of assessment.

B. Cranial nerve function
  1. CN I: olfactory nerve
    a) Assessment: Occlude 1 naris and hold a test tube of mildly aromatic substance (e.g., coffee, peppermint, chocolate, lemon) under the other naris; ask client to identify smell.
    b) Abnormal findings: anosmia (loss of sense of smell), hyposmia (diminished sense of smell)
  2. CN II: optic nerve
    a) Assessment: Check visual acuity, visual fields, pupillary response to light, retinal fields, and optic disc (see section III,E of Chapter 5).
    b) Abnormal findings: visual field defects, absence of either direct or consensual pupillary response to light
  3. CN III, IV, VI: oculomotor, trochlear, and abducens nerves
    a) Assessment: Assess pupils and extraocular movement (see section III,E of Chapter 5).
    b) Abnormal findings: sluggish pupillary response to light or irregular shape, nystagmus, strabismus, ophthalmoplegia (inability to move eyes in specific directions)
  4. CN V: trigeminal nerve
    a) Assessment
      (1) While client's eyes are closed, touch bilateral sites on forehead, cheeks, and jaw with a cotton ball, asking client to state when he/she feels the touch.
      (2) Repeat with sharp object for pain sensation.
      (3) Palpate temporal and masseter muscles as client clenches jaws.
      (4) Test for corneal reflex (see section III,E,6 of Chapter 5).
    b) Abnormal findings: loss of sensation in head, face, or jaw; weakened jaw muscles, evident in deviation of jaw to affected side; absence of corneal reflex
  5. CN VII: facial nerve
    a) Assessment
      (1) Observe as client wrinkles forehead, raises/lowers brows, frowns, smiles with teeth showing, and puffs out cheeks.
      (2) Attempt to open client's tightly closed eyelids.

(3) Test perception of taste.
  (a) Using a pipette or dropper, apply a solution containing a particular type of flavor (salty, sweet, sour, bitter) to 1 area of the tongue at a time.
  (b) Alternate order as different areas are tested, each time asking client to identify the flavor.
  (c) Allow client to rinse mouth with water between tastes.
(4) Although taste in the posterior one-third of the tongue is conveyed by the glossopharyngeal nerve (IX), this area is included as part of the test of facial nerve sensory function.
  b) Abnormal findings: asymmetry, muscle weakness or paralysis, impaired sense of taste
6. CN VIII: acoustic nerve
  a) Assessment: Test hearing (see section III,F of Chapter 5).
  b) Abnormal findings: hearing loss, nystagmus, disturbance of balance, dizziness
7. CN IX, X: glossopharyngeal and vagus nerves
  a) Assessment
    (1) Listen to client's voice for quality.
    (2) Observe soft palate as client says "ah"; soft palate and uvula should rise symmetrically in midline.
    (3) Check gag reflex by touching posterior wall of pharynx with a tongue depressor; palate should rise symmetrically and the pharyngeal muscles should contract.
    (4) Observe swallowing while client drinks a small amount of water (omit if client has no gag reflex).
  b) Abnormal findings: asymmetric response or weak response of palate and uvula, dysphagia, nasal regurgitation, absent gag reflex, hoarseness or nasal-sounding voice
8. CN XI: spinal accessory nerve
  a) Assessment
    (1) Evaluate strength and symmetry of trapezius muscles by asking client to shrug shoulders as you apply resistance.
    (2) Evaluate strength and symmetry of sternocleidomastoid by having client turn head to 1 side and attempt to move chin back to midline as you apply resistance with the palm of your hand; repeat for other side.
  b) Abnormal findings: asymmetry of shoulders, neck, scapulae; muscle weakness; fasciculations; atrophy; paralysis
9. CN XII: hypoglossal nerve
  a) Assessment
    (1) Observe protruded tongue for size, symmetry, and fasciculations.
    (2) Ask client to move the tongue rapidly from side to side, then curl the tongue upward toward the nose and then downward toward the chin.
    (3) Check strength by applying resistance with tongue depressor as client attempts to move depressor to 1 side and then the other.

              (4) Listen to client's ability to pronounce words containing *d, l, n,* or *t.*

        b) Abnormal findings: deviation from midline, atrophy of 1 side or unilateral flaccidity of the tongue, fasciculations, dysarthria

  C. Cerebellar function and the motor system

    1. Assessment

      a) Gait: Observe as bare-footed client walks away and then toward you; gait should be smooth.

      b) Romberg test: While standing close to client, observe ability to maintain balance with eyes closed, feet together, and arms at sides (some swaying is normal); be prepared to protect client from falling.

      c) Tandem walking: Observe as client attempts to walk in straight line in heel-to-toe fashion.

      d) Finger-to-nose test

        (1) Holding up your finger, ask client to touch your finger and then touch his/her own nose.

        (2) Repeat test with increasing speed with your finger at different positions.

        (3) Test both sides.

      e) Heel-to-shin test

        (1) Ask supine client to place heel on opposite knee and then move heel smoothly down shin.

        (2) Test both sides, with eyes open and closed.

      f) Rapid alternating movement

        (1) Ask client to alternate pronation and supination of the hand on the thigh with increasing rapidity.

        (2) Ask client to tap fingers on tabletop or to tap toes on floor as rapidly as possible.

        (3) Ask client to touch each finger to the thumb as rapidly as possible.

    2. Abnormal findings

      a) Gait

        (1) Ataxia: tendency to lose balance, fall to 1 side

        (2) Cerebellar gait: wide, staggering or lurching gait, legs bending at hips

        (3) Parkinsonian gait: stooped posture, arms stiff and unmoving with small shuffling steps

        (4) Steppage (slapping) gait: dragging of feet or lifting them high and bringing them down with a slap on the floor

        (5) Jerky, uncoordinated movements of trunk and neck

b) Positive Romberg sign: inability to maintain balance with eyes closed
c) Leaning or falling toward 1 side during tandem walking
d) Awkwardness and errors during finger-to-nose test
e) Slow, jerky movements or awkwardness during heel-to-shin test
f) Inability/clumsiness during rapid alternating movement tests
g) Nystagmus, particularly with gaze toward side of lesion
h) Cerebellar speech: slow, hesitant, dysarthritic
i) Intention tremors

D. Sensory function
1. General procedure
   a) Have client keep eyes closed during test.
   b) Test each limb distally first; proceed up the limb if sensation is absent or abnormal and determine boundaries of anesthesia or paresthesia.
   c) Minimum test sites include forehead, cheek, hand, lower arm, abdomen, foot, lower leg; compare corresponding sites.
2. Assessment
   a) Light touch: Instruct client to state when skin is touched, while you touch skin lightly with a fine wisp of cotton.
   b) Superficial pain: Instruct client to identify sensation (sharp or dull) as you lightly touch skin with sterile needle (alternating sharp and blunt ends).
   c) Temperature: Instruct client to identify sensation as you alternately touch skin with a test tube full of warm water and a test tube full of cold water.
   d) Vibration: Touch base of a vibrating tuning fork to bony prominences, including clavicles, sternum, wrists, elbows, ankles, knees, and spinous processes; ask client to identify when vibrations start and stop (touch tines of fork to stop vibration).
   e) Position: Hold client's big toe with finger and thumb on either side; move up and down asking client to identify direction of movement; test both feet and repeat with fingers on both hands.
   f) Stereognosis: Place a common object (e.g., key or paper clip) in client's hand and ask client to identify it.
   g) Point localization: Touch client's skin briefly and ask client to open eyes and point to place touched.
   h) Extinction: Touch client simultaneously on corresponding bilateral sites; ask client to state where she/he was touched.
   i) 2-point discrimination: Alternately touch client with 1 or both points of a caliper; assess smallest distance at which client can discern 2 points (closest discrimination is possible on tongue; widest discrimination on back, upper arms, thighs).
   j) Graphesthesia: Have client identify numbers or letters traced with blunt end of pen or pencil on palm or back.

3. Abnormal findings
   a) Anesthesia, hyperesthesia (increased sensitivity to touch), hypesthesia or hypoesthesia (decreased sensitivity to touch), paresthesia (subjective sensations such as numbness or tingling)
   b) Analgesia, hyperalgesia (excessive sensitivity to pain), hypalgesia (diminished sensitivity to pain)
   c) Inability to sense temperature, vibration, or position
   d) Astereognosis (inability to recognize object felt) or inability to recognize numbers or letters traced on skin
   e) Extinction phenomenon (failure to perceive touch on 1 side)

E. Reflexes
   1. Assessment of deep tendon reflexes (DTR)
      a) Biceps (C5, C6)
         (1) Procedure: Have client partially flex arm with palm down; place thumb over biceps tendon and then tap thumb lightly with reflex hammer.
         (2) Normal finding: biceps contraction, elbow flexion
      b) Triceps (C6, C7, C8)
         (1) Procedure: Have client partially flex 1 arm with palm facing inward and arm toward chest; support arm as you tap triceps tendon about 1 inch above elbow.
         (2) Normal finding: extension of elbow, contraction of triceps
      c) Supinator or brachioradialis (C5, C6)
         (1) Procedure: Have client flex arm with palm down and resting on thigh (on abdomen if supine); support arm as you tap styloid process of radius 1–2 inches above wrist.
         (2) Normal finding: flexion of arm and elbow
      d) Patellar (L2, L3, L4)
         (1) Procedure: Have seated client dangle legs; tap patellar tendon.
         (2) Normal finding: extension of knee, contraction of quadriceps
      e) Achilles (S1, S2)
         (1) Procedure: Have seated client dangle legs with ankles dorsiflexed; tap Achilles tendon.
         (2) Normal finding: plantar flexion, then muscle relaxation
   2. Assessment of superficial reflexes
      a) Abdominal (T8–T12)
         (1) Procedure: Stroke each side of the client's abdomen toward midline in each of the 4 quadrants.
         (2) Normal finding: contraction of abdominal muscles and deviation of umbilicus toward the side stroked

b) Anal (S3, S4, S5)
  (1) Procedure: Gently scratch anal region with gloved finger.
  (2) Normal finding: constriction of anal sphincter
c) Cremasteric (male client) (L1, L2)
  (1) Procedure: Gently scratch inner thigh.
  (2) Normal finding: elevation of testicles
d) Plantar (L5, S1, S2)
  (1) Procedure: Stroke sole of client's foot laterally from heel to toes.
  (2) Normal finding: flexion of toes
3. Abnormal findings: pathologic reflexes (in adults, children over 2)
  a) Ankle clonus: Support client's partly flexed knee with 1 hand and use the other to dorsiflex and plantar flex foot several times as client relaxes, then hold foot in sharp dorsiflexion; clonus is a pathologic sign.
  b) Babinski's reflex: dorsiflexion of big toe with or without fanning toes when plantar reflex is assessed
  c) Hoffmann's reflex: Depress distal phalanx of an extended finger and then let go; flexion of thumb or other fingers is positive sign.
  d) Grasp reflex: Place index and middle fingers between client's thumb and index finger and draw them across client's palm; grasping the examiner's fingers is a positive sign.
4. Grading system: Use a stick figure to record tendon reflexes according to the following scale:
  a) Grade 0: absent
  b) Grade +1: diminished but present
  c) Grade +2: normal, average
  d) Grade +3: increased but not necessarily pathologic
  e) Grade +4: hyperactive with clonus

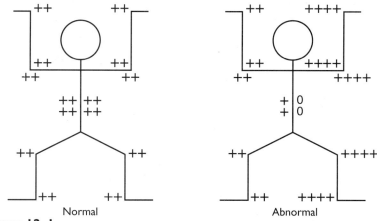

Figure 12–1
Documenting Tendon Reflexes

See text pages

IV. Essential nursing care for client with suspected migraine

A. Nursing assessment
1. Gather relevant health history information (same as section I of this chapter).
2. Perform physical examination to discern signs of brain tumor.

B. Nursing diagnoses
1. Alteration in activities of daily living (ADLs) related to chronic pain
2. Altered role performance related to pain: headaches
3. High risk for injury related to sensory/perceptual alterations involving disturbances of vision
4. Anxiety related to fear of vision loss as expressed by client
5. High risk for noncompliance related to knowledge deficit concerning course and treatment of migraine

C. Nursing implementation (intervention)
1. Educate client about migraine with aura and reassure him/her that visual disturbances are not symptoms of eye disease.
2. Provide information on medication prescribed and tell client that other medications are available if frequency and intensity of attacks are still not controlled.

D. Nursing evaluation
1. Client demonstrates through verbalization an understanding of migraine and aura.
2. Client is able to abort attack by taking medication when aura begins or takes medication on a continual basis to prevent attacks.
3. Client reports he/she is largely free of pain with medication.

1. The nurse has been assigned to complete a full neurologic exam on a 32-year-old male client. He states: "What's taking you so long? It seems like we've been at this for hours." Which of the following is the best response for the nurse to make?

   a. "I understand your frustration. I'm working slowly to make sure I don't miss anything."

   b. "I understand your frustration. A full exam like this one can take a couple of hours. I appreciate your patience."

   c. "Please don't get impatient with me. This exam is what your doctor ordered for you. Perhaps you should talk with her."

   d. "Please don't get impatient with me. I'm doing the best that I can."

2. Which of the following is a true statement about neurologic functioning across the lifespan?

   a. Normal findings among newborns and young infants are different from those of older children.

   b. A child does not reach neurologic maturity until age 7, so assessment should be deferred until that time.

   c. A healthy adult in the middle years does not need routine neurologic screening assessments unless she/he reports some type of problem.

   d. The aging process does not affect neurologic function. The nurse can expect similar findings in all adult clients.

3. A 23-year-old female client with a history of migraines presents to the college health service. She has been experiencing more frequent headaches and they are causing her to miss some classes. She is an excellent student and is planning to graduate soon. In planning care for this client, which of the following nursing diagnoses would be most appropriate?

   a. Alteration in activities of daily living (ADLs) related to pain

   b. Alteration in role performance related to pain

   c. Noncompliance related to knowledge deficit concerning migraine headaches

   d. Ineffective personal coping related to developmental stressors

4. The nurse is assessing a 64-year-old female client who has had a cerebrovascular accident (CVA). The client is exhibiting difficulty with memory and with understanding the meaning of what is said to her. As revealed by these findings, the location of the damage in her brain is the:

   a. Frontal lobe.

   b. Temporal lobe.

   c. Parietal lobe.

   d. Occipital lobe.

5. The nurse is assessing a client who has been diagnosed with Bell's palsy. Which of the following clinical findings is the client most likely to exhibit?

   a. Change in visual acuity

   b. Nystagmus and loss of conjugate extraocular movements

   c. Inability to close the affected eye

   d. Vertigo

6. A parent presents to the emergency room with her 6-month-old male infant who has had a generalized seizure. Which of the following findings would point to meningitis rather than a febrile seizure?

   a. A temperature of 104°F

   b. Irritability

   c. Rapid pulse

   d. A bulging anterior fontanel

7. A 35-year-old male client presents with complaints of severe pain in his lower lip and tongue on the right side of his face. He states that the pain came on suddenly

when he drank cold water earlier in the day. A dysfunction of which of the cranial nerves is most likely to be responsible for his symptoms?

a. Trochlear (IV)
b. Trigeminal (V)
c. Facial (VI)
d. Glossopharyngeal (IX)

8. A 54-year-old male client presents to the clinic with the following symptoms: mild muscle weakness, twitching, and occasional difficulty talking and swallowing. Upon examination the nurse finds some muscle atrophy and spasticity. Which of the following conditions should the nurse suspect?

a. Myasthenia gravis
b. Tetanus infection
c. Amyotrophic lateral sclerosis (ALS)
d. Epilepsy

9. The nurse is performing an assessment on a 62-year-old male client who has been diagnosed with Parkinson's disease. Which of the following findings would the nurse be most likely to observe in this client?

a. Muscle tone that is decreased or even absent
b. Deep tendon reflexes that are hyperactive (+4) coupled with sustained clonus
c. Tremors that are absent at rest but appear with activity
d. A gait in which the trunk is held stiffly and the arms do not swing freely

10. The nurse has just completed a full neurologic assessment of a 58-year-old client. Which of the following findings should the nurse report to the physician?

a. Client has a diminished gag reflex.
b. Client has a positive Romberg test.
c. Client's reflexes are rated at +2.
d. Client has a negative Babinski's reflex.

11. The nurse is assessing the deep tendon reflexes of a 32-year-old female client. The client's arm is resting flexed at the elbow,

palm down. The nurse taps the forearm about 3–5 cm above the wrist on the radial side of the arm. Which of the following is a normal response?

a. Flexion and supination of the forearm and hand
b. Contraction of the biceps muscle
c. Extension of the elbow
d. Sustained clonus of the wrist

12. Which of the following signs are characteristic of upper motor neuron disease rather than lower motor neuron disease?

a. Decreased muscle tone, decreased deep tendon reflexes, absent abdominal reflexes
b. Decreased muscle tone, normal deep tendon reflexes, intention tremors
c. Spastic muscle tone, hyperactive deep tendon reflexes, impaired fine movements
d. Muscle atrophy, absent plantar reflex, fasciculations

ANSWERS

1. **Correct answer is b.** A complete neurologic examination can take 2–3 hours. In this statement the nurse acknowledges the client's feelings, gives him some information, and provides encouragement as well.

   a. While this response acknowledges the client's feelings, it does not provide the client with accurate information about the assessment process. It may also decrease the client's confidence in the abilities of the nurse.
   c. This response minimizes the client's concerns and makes it seem as if the nurse is trying to place blame on the physician.
   d. This response minimizes the client's concerns and sounds angry.

2. **Correct answer is a.** Newborns and young infants display a number of reflexes that disappear during infancy. Absence of or persistence of these reflexes can indicate serious neurologic problems.

b. Although it is true that neurologic maturity is not achieved until the age of 7, this is not a reason to defer an assessment of the system.

c. While it is unlikely that an asymptomatic, healthy adult will require a complete neurologic exam, the nurse should perform a neurologic screening assessment on all clients.

d. Neurologic functioning is greatly affected by the aging process. Some findings considered abnormal in younger clients may be normal in elderly clients.

3. **Correct answer is b.** The client has been missing classes lately because of her headaches. This, for a college student, is an alteration in her role performance. Her role as a student is to attend classes.

   a, c, and **d.** There are not enough data presented to support any of these diagnoses for this client.

4. **Correct answer is b.** The temporal lobe contains the part of the brain responsible for speech comprehension as well as certain aspects of memory. The symptoms described point to damage in this lobe.

   a. The frontal lobe contains the part of the brain responsible for higher thought functions, personality, and social behavior and values. The question reveals no deficits in this area.

   c. The parietal lobe contains the part of the brain responsible for interpretation of sensation and awareness of body parts. The question reveals no deficits in this area.

   d. The occipital lobe contains the part of the brain responsible for interpreting visual stimuli. The question reveals no deficits in this area.

5. **Correct answer is c.** Bell's palsy is a facial dysfunction caused by damage to or paralysis of the facial nerve, cranial nerve VII. A flat nasolabial fold and the inability to raise the eyebrow on the affected side are other signs.

a. A change in visual acuity is not directly related to this condition. Visual problems may be related to dysfunction of the optic nerve, cranial nerve II.

b. Nystagmus and problems with extraocular eye movement are not directly related to this condition. They may be related to dysfunctions of cranial nerves III, IV, or VI.

d. Vertigo is not associated with Bell's palsy but may be caused by a number of other conditions including vestibular neuronitis, Meniere's disease, or a lesion on cranial nerve VIII. Vertigo may also be caused by an adverse reaction to medication.

6. **Correct answer is d.** The nurse should gently palpate the anterior fontanel. A fontanel that is bulging indicates an increase in the infant's intracranial pressure, which would be characteristic of meningitis.

   a, b, and **c.** All of these signs could be characteristic of either an infant with meningitis or one who has just experienced a febrile seizure. None of these findings would help discriminate between the 2 conditions.

7. **Correct answer is b.** This condition is known as tic douloureux, or trigeminal neuralgia. The client experiences stabbing pains along a branch of the trigeminal nerve, in this case, the third branch.

   a. Dysfunction of the trochlear nerve would result in impaired extraocular eye movement.

   c. Dysfunction of the facial nerve would result in facial weakness, asymmetry, or impaired taste sensation in the anterior two-thirds of the tongue.

   d. Dysfunction of the glossopharyngeal nerve would result in pain in the throat or ear, impaired swallowing, or impaired taste sensation in the posterior third of the tongue.

8. **Correct answer is c.** Progressive muscle weakness, twitching, atrophy, and spasticity are characteristic of this disease. The difficulty in talking and swallowing could indicate a weakness in the musculature supplied by the cranial nerves. In addition, the client's age is a key factor. ALS generally affects clients in their 50s and 60s.

   a. Symptoms of this disease include extreme, not mild, muscle weakness. Cranial nerves may be affected, but the first to be affected are usually those with ocular function. Spasticity and twitching are not found.
   b. Tetanus infection can cause spasticity of muscles, especially of mastication. None of the other symptoms or signs described here, however, are typical.
   d. None of these symptoms or signs is indicative of epilepsy, which is characterized by seizures.

9. **Correct answer is d.** This is an accurate description of the typical gait of a client with Parkinson's disease. Destruction of neurons in the basal ganglia causes these and other abnormalities.

   a. Muscle tone in the client with Parkinson's disease is increased, not decreased. This finding would be consistent with lower motor neuron or cerebellar disorders.
   b. Deep tendon reflexes in the client with Parkinson's disease are not hyperactive. This finding would be consistent with upper motor neuron disorders.

   c. The client with Parkinson's disease exhibits resting tremors. Intention tremors, which are described here, are found in cerebellar disorders.

10. **Correct answer is b.** A positive Romberg test, in which the patient cannot stand steadily with eyes closed, indicates the client has sensory ataxia, in which position sense is lost.

    a. While this may be a cause for concern, normal clients can have a diminished or absent gag reflex.
    c. This is a normal finding.
    d. This is a normal finding. A positive Babinski's reflex is normal in infants.

11. **Correct answer is a.** This is the normal response to the eliciting of the supinator (brachioradialis) reflex, described here.

    b. This is a normal response to the eliciting of the biceps reflex, in which the biceps tendon is struck above the elbow.
    c. This is a normal response to the eliciting of the triceps reflex, in which the triceps tendon is struck above the elbow.
    d. Sustained clonus is never a normal response.

12. **Correct answer is c.** These are some of the clinical manifestations of upper motor neuron disease.

    a and d. These are some of the clinical manifestations of lower motor neuron disease.
    b. These are some of the clinical manifestations of cerebellar dysfunction.

Health Assessment Comprehensive Review Questions

1. A thorough health history provides the following information:

   a. Personal data about the nurse interviewer
   b. Data for a temporary chart, destroyed after the client moves away
   c. Baseline physical examination data
   d. Data for development of nursing diagnoses for the client

2. The client, a 55-year-old diabetic male, complains of pain in his calves when walking. Which is the best question to ask that will directly investigate this client's chief complaint?

   a. "The pain isn't keeping you from performing your normal activities, is it?"
   b. "When were you first diagnosed with diabetes?"
   c. "Have you found anything that relieves the pain?"
   d. "Do you have any allergies?"

3. The best assessment technique to determine temperature of a body area is:

   a. Inspection of all body areas to compare color.
   b. Palpation with the fingertips.
   c. Palpation with the dorsal surface of the hand.
   d. Bimanual palpation.

4. Mental health assessment is a process that is best performed during:

   a. One session.
   b. The initial health history interview.
   c. Multiple sessions.
   d. The physical assessment.

5. Which of the following is a normal finding within the cardiovascular system of a child?

   a. Wide, paradoxical splitting of S_2 (second heart sound)
   b. Diastolic murmur
   c. Diminished femoral pulses
   d. Venous hum

6. While working in a nursing home, the nurse sees a newly admitted 86-year-old client who has recently lost her husband of 63 years. Her family lives more than 120 miles away. The nurse assesses this client's mental health status, noting that she has not eaten much in the last week. The client has refused to meet the other residents and prefers to stay in bed all day. The nurse's *priority* concern about this client is:

   a. She is showing symptoms of depression.
   b. She is planning suicide.
   c. She has no visitors.
   d. She has not adjusted to the nursing home routine.

7. When examining the client, a 33-year-old black male who has relapses of active hepatitis B, the nurse notices that his sclerae are a pale yellow. However, since dark-skinned persons may normally have a yellowish cast to their sclerae, what other body area should the nurse check for a yellow discoloration?

   a. Fingernails
   b. Scalp
   c. Hard palate
   d. Skin behind the ears

8. A 4-year-old boy comes to the pediatric clinic with many different types of pruritic skin lesions all over his body. There are red

papules, vesicles, excoriations, and crusts. He is afebrile, but his mother reports he had a temperature of 100°F 4 days ago, the evening before the lesions appeared. These clinical findings are indicative of:

a. Varicella (chicken pox).
b. Rubella (German measles).
c. Poison ivy.
d. Shingles.

9. Which of the following is the most important role of the nurse in preventing deaths from skin cancer, particularly malignant melanoma?

a. Teaching self-assessment of the skin
b. Teaching people to limit the time they spend sunbathing
c. Recommending the use of 100% cotton clothing
d. Teaching clients the American Cancer Society's 8 warning signs of cancer

10. The nurse is examining a 3-month-old male infant. His mother has reported that he has been vomiting for 24 hours. Which of the following would be an important physical finding that relates directly to the mother's concerns?

a. The diaper the infant is wearing is dry.
b. The infant is not able to raise his body on his hands when lying prone.
c. The infant's anterior fontanel is sunken.
d. There is a greenish discharge from the infant's nose.

11. The nurse is completing a health history of a 50-year-old male client. The client tells the nurse that he has noticed a decrease in his sense of taste and that "everything seems to taste the same." Which of the following would be the best response for the nurse to make?

a. "Your decreased sense of taste is probably caused by the effects of aging. As people get older their senses lose some acuity."
b. "Do you smoke? Smoking destroys the olfactory receptors in the mouth."

c. "When I am done with your history I'll do a physical exam. I'll be sure to test your olfactory and facial nerves at that time."
d. "This is unusual. I'm going to refer you to a specialist."

12. Which of the following is a major cause of lung disease in children?

a. Asthma
b. Tuberculosis
c. Lung cancer
d. Secondhand smoke

13. The nurse is auscultating the chest of a 43-year-old male client for breath sounds. The client has no respiratory complaints. Which of the following is the correct technique for the nurse to use?

a. The nurse should listen to all sites on the anterior thorax, all sites on the posterior thorax, all sites on the right lateral thorax, and finally all sites on the left lateral thorax.
b. The nurse should auscultate the anterior thorax, listening to the sites first on the right side and then on the left side. The nurse should repeat the procedure for the posterior thorax and then for the right and left lateral thorax.
c. The nurse should listen to all sites on the right anterior thorax, then to the right posterior thorax. The nurse should repeat the procedure for the left anterior and posterior thorax and then for the right and left lateral thorax.
d. The nurse should listen to 1 auscultatory site on the right anterior thorax and then to the corresponding site on the left anterior thorax. The nurse should repeat this procedure for all auscultatory sites on the anterior, posterior, and right and left lateral thorax.

14. The nurse obtains all of the following data about a pregnant 36-year-old woman. Which

piece of data should be reported to the physician immediately?

a. Her blood pressure is 138/86 and her pulse is 90.

b. She has a heart murmur audible along the left sternal border.

c. Her ankles have evidence of non-pitting edema.

d. She experiences some dizziness when changing positions.

15. The physician has left orders for the nurse to do a cardiovascular assessment for a 6-month-old client. Which of the following orders should the nurse question?

a. Complete cardiovascular workup including electrocardiogram (ECG) and serum electrolytes

b. Complete cardiovascular workup including developmental assessment

c. Complete cardiovascular workup including echocardiogram

d. Complete cardiovascular workup including ECG and electroencephalogram (EEG)

16. The nurse offers to teach breast self-examination to the client, age 60. The client says, "I'm too old for this. Besides, I feel funny about touching my breasts." The best nursing action is to:

a. Give her written materials and a video to practice at home.

b. Encourage her to get a mammogram every 6 months instead.

c. Explore her feelings about breast self-examination before teaching her the technique.

d. Emphasize that the risk of breast cancer increases with age, that no one is ever too old to learn, and that she should not "feel funny" about examining her breasts.

17. Which of the following findings would support a diagnosis of cholecystitis?

a. A positive Rovsing's sign

b. A positive Murphy's sign

c. A negative psoas sign

d. A negative obturator sign

18. A 36-year-old female client has been diagnosed with diverticulitis. She states, "I hate fruits and vegetables. I can't follow a diet like that!" Which of the following nursing diagnoses would be most appropriate for this client?

a. Altered nutrition, less than body requirements, related to abdominal pain

b. Colonic constipation related to inadequate dietary intake of fiber

c. High risk for altered health maintenance related to potential noncompliance with dietary restrictions

d. High risk for impaired individual coping related to chronic illness

19. The nurse is interviewing a 61-year-old female client. The client describes herself as generally healthy and active. Lately, however, she has had some pain in her wrists and hands. To help establish a diagnosis of arthritis, which of the following actions should the nurse take first?

a. Assess the client's joints for deformity, function, and range of motion.

b. Obtain a detailed family history, focusing on musculoskeletal disorders.

c. Obtain a full medication history, focusing on medications with musculoskeletal effects.

d. Inspect the client's hip and knee joints, and observe the client's gait.

20. A complete assessment of the client described in the previous question reveals joint degeneration. Which of the following nursing diagnoses would be most appropriate?

a. Impaired physical mobility related to limited joint movement secondary to aging

b. Self-care deficits related to joint degeneration secondary to aging.

c. Acute pain related to joint degeneration

d. Ineffective coping related to actual or perceived lifestyle changes secondary to arthritis

21. The nurse is taking a health history of a 37-year-old client who has been diagnosed with chronic prostatitis. Which of these statements indicates the client's need for further education?

   a. "Whenever I have an acute infection, I know that I have to take all my medication to make sure the infection is completely gone."
   b. "I'm glad I don't have any special dietary restrictions to adhere to."
   c. "To be more comfortable, I should avoid sitting for long periods of time."
   d. "I should avoid sexual intercourse during an acute infection, but otherwise it's OK."

22. A 21-year-old client presents to the college health service with a concern about amenorrhea. She is an active and healthy woman and enjoys long-distance running. She states: "I did one of those home pregnancy tests. It was negative, but I still think I may be pregnant since my period hasn't come." Which of the following is the best first response for the nurse to make?

   a. "I'll perform another pregnancy test. Amenorrhea is almost always related to pregnancy. Have you had unprotected intercourse in the last month?"
   b. "Amenorrhea in a woman your age for reasons other than pregnancy is very unusual. Let's talk about the options you have for this pregnancy."
   c. "It is not unusual for women who are engaged in strenuous physical activity to experience amenorrhea. Tell me about your training program and your diet."
   d. "It is not unusual for women who are suffering from emotional upset to have amenorrhea. Are you experiencing any unusual stresses?"

23. A client has come to the clinic with a concern about headaches. She states: "I have them every day. I'm sure it is something awful like a brain tumor. That's what my grandmother died from." Which of the

following is the best response for the nurse to make?

   a. "Having headaches does not mean you have a brain tumor. Everyone has headaches at one time or another."
   b. "Do you have any other symptoms along with your headaches? Without other symptoms, a brain tumor is very unlikely."
   c. "I understand your concern. I'm going to refer you to a specialist for a complete neurologic assessment."
   d. "I understand your concern, particularly with your family history. Let's begin by getting more information about your symptoms."

24. While assessing a 68-year-old male client, the nurse notes his wide-based, lurching gait. The client cannot stand steadily with his eyes either open or closed. He also exhibits intention tremors. These findings are most consistent with:

   a. Parkinson's disease.
   b. Muscular dystrophy.
   c. Cerebellar ataxia.
   d. Sensory ataxia.

ANSWERS

1. Correct answer is d. Significant nursing diagnoses can be based on the health history alone or in combination with physical assessment data.

   a. The nurse interviewer may share some personal data as a means of building rapport during the interview, but the inclusion of personal data in the client's health history is inappropriate.
   b. The health history provides data for a confidential, permanent, chronologic, and legal record.
   c. Baseline physical examination data are objective data collected to compare with future physical examination data to detect significant changes and health deviations. They are not part of the health history.

2. **Correct answer is c.** The nurse must ask about aggravating and alleviating factors as part of her full assessment of the client's chief complaint.

   a. The nurse is asking a leading question to which the client may not respond accurately.
   b. The initial diagnosis of diabetes is important health history information, but is not the best question to ask to investigate directly the chief complaint of pain in calves when walking.
   d. Information about allergies is essential for a complete health history, but it is not directly related to investigating this chief complaint.

3. **Correct answer is c.** The dorsal surface of the hand is more sensitive to temperature than other parts of the hand.

   a. Temperature is assessed by palpation, not inspection.
   b. Fingertips are used to assess pulsations. The temperature in the fingertips of the examiner may interfere with accurate temperature assessment of the client.
   d. Bimanual palpation is using both hands to palpate deeply or to feel an object between the hands.

4. **Correct answer is c.** Because mental health assessment is a continual process, multiple sessions are necessary for an accurate assessment.

   a. Completion of a mental health assessment is impossible in just 1 session.
   b and d. Some data relevant to the mental health assessment may be collected during the initial health history interview and the physical assessment, but this does not comprise a complete assessment.

5. **Correct answer is d.** A venous hum is common in children. It is heard in both systole and diastole over the veins at the base of the neck.

   a. Wide, paradoxical splitting of S_2, or splitting on expiration, is an abnormal finding.

Splitting of S_2 on inspiration is a common, normal finding in children.
   b. A diastolic murmur is probably an abnormal finding. A systolic, functional murmur occurs in 50% of children and most often is a normal finding if there is no other evidence of cardiovascular disease.
   c. Diminished femoral pulses are an abnormal finding and may indicate a cardiac defect, such as coarctation of the aorta.

6. **Correct answer is a.** Loss of appetite, tiredness, fatigue, and decreased social interaction are some of the signs of depression.

   b. These symptoms alone do not indicate she is planning suicide.
   c. This is a cause for concern, but not the priority concern. Lack of visits from family and friends is a problem that may be contributing to her depression.
   d. The elderly as well as the general population have difficulty adjusting to a major lifestyle change. This may be as a result of her depression, which is the nurse's priority concern.

7. **Correct answer is c.** During episodes of active hepatitis, the posterior portion of the hard palate may also exhibit a yellow pigmentation.

   a. Yellow fingernails may occur with aging, nicotine staining, or lymphatic or thyroid abnormalities.
   b and d. A yellowish cast does not become evident in the scalp or skin of dark-skinned persons.

8. **Correct answer is a.** Varicella characteristically exhibits a mild fever before eruption of pruritic papules, vesicles, excoriations, and crusts.

   b. Rubella exhibits erythematous macules.
   c. The plant poison ivy causes a contact dermatitis of red vesicles with no prodromal fever.
   d. Shingles exhibits skin lesions similar to varicella but usually occurs in older persons. Lesions do not erupt all over the body but follow peripheral nerve routes.

9. Correct answer is a. Skin self-assessment can be lifesaving to a client; he/she can monitor any changes in moles and seek health care immediately. A yearly skin exam by a health professional is also recommended.

b. There is no safe level of sun exposure. The nurse should not encourage any level of sun tanning.
c. The use of 100% cotton clothing alone will not protect the skin. Clothes should cover all exposed body areas and should not allow UV light penetration.
d. This is a very useful nursing action but it is secondary to teaching skin self-assessment where the goal is preventing deaths from skin cancer.

10. Correct answer is c. Because of the infant's history and age, the nurse should be concerned about dehydration. Of the choices provided, this is the only clear indicator of dehydration.

a. Decreased urine output is a sign of dehydration, but the nurse does not have enough information to know if this finding is significant; the infant's mother, for example, may just have changed the diaper.
b. This is a reflection of growth and development rather than hydration status and is not an unusual finding in an infant of this age.
d. Such a discharge may indicate an upper respiratory infection but is not an indicator of dehydration.

11. Correct answer is c. The nurse will gather more data about the client's complaint during the exam by testing the client's olfactory and facial nerves, cranial nerves that are responsible for taste sensations.

a. While the olfactory sense may be affected by age in some clients, the nurse does not have enough data to make this statement in this situation.
b. While smoking does affect the sense of taste, there is no such thing as an olfactory receptor in the mouth.
d. The nurse does not have enough data to make a referral at this time.

12. Correct answer is d. Research has consistently supported the finding that secondhand smoke, or passive smoking, increases the incidence of upper respiratory infections, bronchitis, and asthma in children.

a, b, and **c.** Asthma, tuberculosis, and lung cancer are lung diseases. Exposure to secondhand smoke can increase a child's susceptibility to all lung diseases.

13. Correct answer is d. The front, back, and sides of the chest must be auscultated contralaterally. Each auscultatory site must be compared to its corresponding site on the opposite side of the chest to compare the quality of breath sounds. Otherwise, abnormalities that are difficult to hear, such as diminished breath sounds, may be missed.

a, b, and **c.** Using these techniques it is impossible to compare breath sounds at right and left corresponding auscultatory sites.

14. Correct answer is b. The increased blood flow associated with pregnancy can cause innocent murmurs. Any murmur, however, requires further assessment. This finding should be reported to the physician without delay.

a. These vital signs are within normal limits for this client.
c and **d.** These findings are not unusual in a pregnant woman.

15. Correct answer is d. The nurse should question the need for an EEG during a complete cardiovascular workup.

a. An ECG and serum electrolytes test may be part of a cardiovascular workup. The ECG results show the electrical activity of the heart. The serum electrolytes results may reveal electrolyte imbalances with cardiac manifestations.
b. A developmental assessment would give information about this child's rate of growth and development.
c. A echocardiagram will assess the structure and mobility of the infant's heart and may reveal congenital defects.

16. Correct answer is c. Giving the client an opportunity to talk through her concerns about breast self-examination will increase her self-awareness. She may gain insight into her behavior, feel more comfortable with her body, and comply with breast self-exams because it is her choice.

a. Written materials and a video are appropriate as a follow-up but are not a substitute for personal, one-on-one teaching.
b. In her age group, a yearly mammogram is recommended in addition to a clinical examination.
d. This response invalidates her feelings and may increase her anxiety.

17. Correct answer is b. This finding, of increased tenderness and stopped inspiration when the examiner places her/his fingers deep beneath the right costal margin, suggests a diagnosis of acute cholecystitis.

a. A positive Rovsing's sign of referred rebound tenderness in the right lower quadrant when pressure is applied in the left lower quadrant suggests appendicitis.
c. A negative psoas sign, in which abdominal pain is not increased when the client raises the thigh against the pressure of the examiner's hand, suggests that appendicitis is not present. Furthermore, it does not give any data about possible cholecystitis.
d. A negative obturator sign, in which there is no right hypogastric pain when the examiner flexes the right hip and knee and rotates the leg internally, suggests that appendicitis is not present. Furthermore, it does not give any data about possible cholecystitis.

18. Correct answer is c. The client's statement reveals that she hates the foods on her recommended diet and feels that she cannot follow it. This puts her at high risk for altered health maintenance.

a. There is not enough data to support this nursing diagnosis. The client could avoid fruits and vegetables and still ingest more than her body's requirements of nutrients and calories.

b. The client may well experience colonic constipation if she does not follow the recommended diet, but that has not yet occurred.
d. There is not sufficient evidence to support a diagnosis that the client is experiencing impaired individual coping in relation to her illness.

19. Correct answer is a. The nurse should start with an assessment of the client's current health. Getting more information about the client's actual abilities and limitations would begin this process.

b and **c.** Although both of these should be included in a full assessment of the client, neither would be the place for the nurse to begin.
d. Inspection of these joints, as well as all others, and observation of the client's gait would give the nurse additional information. This would not, however, be the place for the nurse to begin.

20. Correct answer is c. The client has described pain. Based on her description of the pain and her general comments about her health status it is most likely that a diagnosis of arthritis will be confirmed.

a. Although this is a concern and can be a complication related to arthritis, the nurse does not have enough information to assign this diagnosis.
b. The nurse does not have enough information about this client to assign this diagnosis.
d. Based on the way the client presented herself to the nurse, this will probably be a concern. She will most likely have some alteration in her lifestyle secondary to this diagnosis, but the nurse does not yet have enough information to assign this diagnosis.

21. Correct answer is b. It is recommended that men with prostatitis avoid foods and beverages that have a diuretic action or increase prostatic secretions, including drinks containing caffeine or alcohol as well as foods containing certain spices.

a. This statement indicates the client understands the need to complete the course of oral antibiotics.

c. This statement indicates an understanding of the possible link between long sedentary periods and prostate inflammation.

d. This statement indicates that the client understands the need to avoid sexual intercourse during the acute inflammation but that intercourse can be beneficial after that to discourage the retention of prostatic fluids.

22. **Correct answer is c.** Amenorrhea sometimes occurs in women who participate in strenuous physical activity, such as long-distance running, or when they lose weight suddenly. The nurse must start by gathering more data about this client. This response sets the stage for the interview.

   a. The nurse must certainly rule out pregnancy, but amenorrhea can occur as a result of other causes. The nurse's question may be necessary later on, but should not be her first response.

   b. The nurse is making the assumption that this client is pregnant. She should gather additional data before talking with the client about her pregnancy options.

   d. Although emotional upset can cause menstrual irregularity, the nurse should not assume this is the cause in light of the other data she has about the client. Later in the interview she may want to explore stresses present in the client's life.

23. **Correct answer is d.** With this comment the nurse has validated the client's feelings and has set the stage for working with the client to address her concerns.

   a. This response minimizes the client's concerns and dismisses her symptoms.

   b. This response alludes to the need to get more information but minimizes the client's concerns in the process.

   c. The nurse has validated the client's concern but does not yet have enough information to determine the need to refer the client to a specialist.

24. **Correct answer is c.** These findings are indicative of cerebellar ataxia.

   a. Clients with Parkinson's disease display a shuffling gait in which the trunk is held rigidly. Their steps hardly clear the ground, and their tremors occur at rest.

   b. Clients with muscular dystrophy exhibit a waddling or rolling gait. One hip is elevated while the other is depressed.

   d. Clients with sensory ataxia cannot stand steadily with their eyes closed but can do so with their eyes open. When walking, they throw their feet forward and outward.